TARGET JIPMER

(Model Questions with Solved Explanatory Answers)

"Get the inside edge! Authored by Jipmerites"

MAY 2019 (Supplement)

Dr. T. ARUN BABU
MD Pediatrics (JIPMER), DAA (CMC, Vellore), MBA (HM)
Fellow in Neonatal Perinatal Medicine (Canada)
Associate Professor and Head, Department of Pediatrics
All India Institute of Medical Sciences (AIIMS)
Mangalagiri, Andhra Pradesh
Puducherry – 605009
Website: www.drarunbabu.in

Peepee Publishers and Distributors (P) Ltd.®

TARGET JIPMER MAY 2019 (Supplement)

Published by
Pawaninder P. Vij and Anupam Vij

Peepee Publishers and Distributors (P) Ltd.
Head Office: 160, Shakti Vihar, Pitam Pura, Delhi-110 034 (India)

Correspondence Address:

7/31, First Floor, Ansari Road, Daryaganj
New Delhi-110 002 (India)

Ph: 41512412, 23246245, 9811156083

e-mail: peepee160@yahoo.co.in

e-mail: peepee160@gmail.com

www.peepeepub.com

join us on facebook.com/pp.publishers

First Edition: 2020

ISBN: 978-81-8445-274-7

Dedication

To my Parents, Teachers,
my wife Dr. Sharmila,
my kids Akshaya and Akash

Disclaimer:

This book fully complies with the non-disclosure agreement (NDA) levied by JIPMER. This book contains Model questions with solved explanatory answers. No questions included in this book have been obtained from any candidates registered for JIPMER exam. Any resemblance to the original JIPMER questions, if present, is purely coincidental. The author, contributors, publisher or sellers cannot be held responsible for any damage or loss caused to anyone, directly or indirectly.

PREFACE

We are very happy in bringing out yet another supplement of TARGET JIPMER book. Big thanks for making TARGET JIPMER series the best book for JIPMER PGMEE preparation. This book series was started with the sole purpose of making model JIPMER questions accessible to PG aspirants. The questions have been solved by a team of subject experts from reputed academic backgrounds. This book is tailor made for JIPMER PG entrance exam preparation. Most of our contributors are JIPMER alumni and have personally written JIPMER PG exams in the last few years and are well experienced and aware of the examination pattern. JIPMER questions are mostly taken from standard textbooks and articles. Though the pattern of JIPMER questions have changed in the last few years, the high yield area remains the same. You will understand this after going through all the volumes of 4th edition of TARGET JIPMER.

We have incorporated a systematic approach in solving each and every question which can be appreciated while reading this book. The schematic diagrams, tables, illustrations, bulleted key points and references are the highlights of this book and will make reading and understanding of the material easier and effective. Every solved question will have a valid reference citing a standard textbook or article in order to increase the credibility of the answers. The focused explanations should help you solve questions from same topics in the future easily.

I would like to thank all the contributors for their commitment and hard work that has led to the tremendous success of this book series. I wish to thank our publishers, Mr. Pawaninder Pal Vij and Mr. Anupam Vij, the Directors of Peepee Publishers and Distributors (P) Ltd, who have always been a pillar of support to our team. I would also like to thank our publishing team for their relentless efforts in releasing this book in a short notice. I am deeply indebted to students for their overwhelming support, feedback and critical appraisal. We are looking forward to hear your feedback and are fully committed in bringing out better editions in the future. For JIPMER students, a JIPMERITE tag is a matter of pride which they carry as a badge of honour throughout their professional life. For most others it is a dream. I believe and hope that this book will make your dream come true.

All the best!

T. Arun Babu

Website: *www.drarunbabu.in*

Email: *babuarun.t@gmail.com*

"Books are infinite in number and time is short. The secret of knowledge is to take what is essential."

–Swami Vivekananda

CONTRIBUTORS

Dr. Arun Babu T, MD Pediatrics (JIPMER), DAA (CMC), Fellow NPM (Canada)
Associate Professor, Department of Pediatrics
Indira Gandhi Medical College and Research Institute (IGMC&RI)
Puducherry – 605 009
(Chief Editor)

Dr. Arundhathi S, MD Pathology
Associate Professor, Department of Pathology
All India Institute of Medical Sciences (AIIMS)
Mangalagiri – 522 503
(Pathology)

Dr. Arul Varman, MD Psychiatry (JIPMER)
Assistant Professor, Department of Psychiatry
Indira Gandhi Medical College and Research Institute (IGMC&RI)
Puducherry – 605 009
(Psychiatry)

Dr. Dinesh Kumar, MD Pediatrics
Assistant Professor, Department of Pediatrics
Indira Gandhi Medical College and Research Institute (IGMC&RI)
Puducherry – 605 009
(Pediatrics)

Dr. Jean Fredrick, MD Physiology
Assistant Professor
Department of Physiology
Mahatma Gandhi Medical College and Research Institute (MGMC&RI), Pillaiyarkuppam
Puducherry
(Physiology)

Dr. Madhav Rao, MD Pharm (JIPMER)
Associate Professor, Department of Pharmacology
All India Institute of Medical Sciences (AIIMS)
Mangalagiri – 522 503
(Pharmacology)

Dr. Mugunthan N, MS Anatomy, DNB, PhD, MBA
Professor of Anatomy
Sree Mookambika Institute of Medical Sciences
Kulasekaram, Kanyakumari District
Tamil Nadu – 629 161
(Anatomy)

Dr. Mukul Mohindra, MS (Ortho), DNB, MNAMS, Dip.SICOT (Belgium)
Fellow National Board (Arthroscopy and Sports Medicine)
Sports Injury Center, Safdarjung Hospital and VMM College
New Delhi
(Orthopaedics)

Dr. Prasanna S, MD Microbiology (AFMC, Pune)
Assistant Professor, Department of Microbiology
Shri Sathya Sai Medical College and Research institute
Kancheepuram
Tamil Nadu – 603 108
(Microbiology)

Dr. Priyanka Choudhary, MD Community Medicine
Senior Resident, Department of Community Medicine
PGIMS, Rohtak, Haryana
(Preventive and Social Medicine)

Dr. Prudhvinath Reddy A, MD, DNB, Fellow in Body Imaging
Assistant Professor, Department of Radiodiagnosis
All India Institute of Medical Sciences (AIIMS)
Mangalagiri – 522 503
(Radiology)

Dr. R Rajamahendran, MS, MRCS (UK), FMAS, MCh (SGE)
Assistant Professor in Surgical Gastroenterology
GVMCH, Villupuram, Tamil Nadu
Consultant Surgical Gastroenterologist and Advanced Lap GI Surgeon
RRM Gastro Surgical and Research Centre, Villupuram
Director, "KONCPT NEET" Medical Coaching Centre
(Surgery)

Dr. Ranjith AR, MD Pathology (JIPMER)
Molecular Pathologist, Bangalore
(Pathology)

Dr. Sangeeta Dhanger, DA, DNB, MNAMS
Assistant Professor, Department of Anesthesiology
Indira Gandhi Medical College and Research Institute (IGMC&RI)
Puducherry – 605 009
(Anesthesiology)

Dr. Satvinder Singh Bakshi, MS ENT (JIPMER), DNB
Associate Professor, Department of Otorhinolaryngology
All India Institute of Medical Sciences (AIIMS)
Mangalagiri, Andhra Pradesh
(ENT)

Dr. Sharmila Arun Babu, MS OBG (JIPMER)
Assistant Professor, Department of OBG
Indira Gandhi Medical College and Research Institute (IGMC&RI)
Puducherry – 605 009
(OBG)

Dr. Sindhujha Sekar G, JIPMER, DGO, DNB OG
Assistant Professor
Department of OBG
Sri Venkateswara Medical College Hospital and Research Centre, Puducherry
(OBG)

Dr. Soumya Sathyan, MD General Medicine
Senior Resident
MES Medical College, Perintalmanna
(Medicine)

Dr. Udayashankar C, MD Dermatology (JIPMER), MBA (HM)
Professor and Head
Department of Dermatology
Indira Gandhi Medical College and Research Institute
(IGMC&RI)
Puducherry - 605 009
(Dermatology)

Dr. Usha S Adiga, MBBS MD PhD
Professor, Department of Biochemistry
KS Hegde Medical Academy
Mangalore, Karnataka
(Biochemistry)

Dr. Venipriya, MS Ophthalmology
Senior Resident, Department of Ophthalmology
Indira Gandhi Medical College and Research Institute
(IGMC&RI)
Puducherry - 605 009
(Ophthalmology)

Dr. Vinoth Kumar S, MD General Medicine
Assistant Professor, Department of General Medicine
Indira Gandhi Medical College and Research Institute
(IGMC&RI)
Puducherry - 605 009
(General Medicine)

Dr. Yatiraj Singi, MD Forensic Medicine
Professor, Department of Forensic Medicine
Sree Mookambika Institute of Medical Sciences
Kulasekharam, Dist Kanya Kumari, TN
(Forensic Medicine)

ACKNOWLEDGEMENTS

Target JIPMER – Previous Edition Contributors

Dr. Bharath Kumar V D, MD Assistant Professor of Pharmacology, BGSGIMS, Bangalore, Karnataka.

Dr. Abhishek Bhaumik, MS Senior Resident, Department of Surgery, West Bengal HS.

Dr. Kantamani Bala Teja, MS (ENT) MCH Head and Neck Surgery Senior Resident, Mumbai.

Dr. Nishanth Sampath, MD Clinical Neurophysiologist, SIMS, Chennai, Tamil Nadu.

Dr. Suthanthira Kannan, MD Assistant Professor of Community Medicine, ESI Medical College, Hyderabad.

Dr. Pratheep, MS General Surgery MCH Oncosurgery Resident.

Dr. Balamurugan N, DCH, DNB, MRCPCH, Assistant Professor, Department of Pediatrics, SLIMS, Puducherry.

Dr.Tejswita Rajpal Hande, MBBS, DGO, MUHS, Nashik.

Dr. Saranya K, MD Physio (JIPMER), Assistant Professor of Physiology, JIPMER, Puducherry.

Dr. Abarna Devi S, DDVL (JIPMER), MD Medicine, Assistant Professor of Medicine, ESIMC, Chennai.

Dr. Anshu Bahl, MD Anatomy (AIIMS), New Delhi.

Dr. Ankit Agarwal, MD RT (JIPMER), Senior Resident, GMCH, Sector 32, Chandigarh.

Dr. Naga Dharshan Devendra, MD (JIPMER), Associate Professor and Course Director, Department of Biochemistry and Genetics, Trinity School of Medicine, Saint Vincent and Grenadines.

Dr. Saseendar S, MS (Ortho), DNB, Dip SICOT (Belgium), MNAMS, Care Sports Injury, Chennai.

Dr. Srirangaraj S, MD, Professor, Department of Microbiology, MGMCRI, Puducherry.

Dr. Sri Vengadesh Gopal, MS (JIPMER), Assistant Professor, Department of Surgery, IGMC and RI, Puducherry.

Dr. Sumanth MM, MD (JIPMER), DNB, Associate Professor of Community Medicine, MMC and RI, Mysore, Karnataka.

Dr. Sentitoshi, MD (JIPMER) Forensic Medicine, Former Assistant Professor, MGMC and RI, Puducherry.

Dr. Asayas Bosco Chandrakumar, MS, Associate Professor of Surgery, SLIMS, Puducherry.

Dr. Mahesh Nagappa, MD Anaes (JIPMER), DNB, MNAMS, Assistant Professor, SLIMS, Puducherry.

Dr. Sinhasan SP, MD, Associate Professor of Pathology, IGMC and RI, Puducherry.

Dr. Amiya Kumar Nath, MD (JIPMER), Associate Professor of Dermatology, IGMC and RI, Puducherry.

Dr. Venkateswaran R, MD, Associate Professor of Medicine, JIPMER, Puducherry.

Dr. Niranjan G, MD Biochem (JIPMER), Associate Professor of Biochemistry, AIIMS, Nagpur.

Dr. VishnuKanth, MD (JIPMER), Associate Professor, Department of Respiratory Medicine, JIPMER, Puducherry.

Dr. Dilli Kumar, MD (JIPMER), Associate Professor of Pediatrics, JIPMER, Puducherry.

Dr. Dilip Kumar R, MD (JIPMER), MRCP (UK), Dr. Mehta's Hospitals, Chetpet, Chennai-31.

Dr. Sachidananda Adiga, MD, Professor of Pharmacology, KS Hegde Medical Academy, Mangalore.

Dr. Giriyanna Gowda, MD, Associate Professor of Community Medicine, KIMS, Bangalore, Karnataka.

Dr. Gomathi Shankar V, MS (JIPMER), DNB, MNAMS, Associate Professor of Surgery, JIPMER, Puducherry.

Dr. Karthik, MD Physiology (JIPMER), Associate Professor of Physiology, JIPMER, Puducherry.

Dr. Lourdu Jafrin, MD, Associate Professor of Pharmacology, IGMC and RI, Puducherry.

Dr. Mahalakshmy T, MD PSM (JIPMER), Associate Professor of PSM, JIPMER, Puducherry.

Dr. Melvin George, MD, DM Clin Pharm (JIPMER), Assistant Professor, Cardiac Clinical Trials and Research, Department of Cardiology, SRM Medical College and Hospital, Potheri, Tamil Nadu.

Dr. Naveen Nair, MS Orthopedics (JIPMER), Associate Professor of Orthopedics, IGMC and RI, Puducherry.

Dr. Noyal Mariya Joseph, MD (JIPMER), Associate Professor of Microbiology, JIPMER, Puducherry.

Dr. Raveendranath, MS Anatomy (St Johns), Associate Professor of Anatomy, JIPMER, Puducherry.

Dr. Rupa Vani, DNB, Assistant Professor of Obstetrics and Gynecology, IGMC and RI, Puducherry.

Sincere Thanks to:

Dr. Nivedhan, MBBS, Stanley Medical College, Chennai.
Dr. Anoop Singh, MBBS, HIMS, Hassan.
Dr. Nadim Anjum, MBBS, North Bengal Medical College, Siliguri, West Bengal.
Dr. Mimi Janet, MBBS, Velammal Medical College, Madurai.
Dr. Abdul Hazan, MD (Physician) Russia, Rostov State Medical University.
Dr. Allan Deepak, MBBS, Thoothukudi Medical College, Tamil Nadu.
Dr. Arunima Das, MBBS, Midnapore Medical College, Paschim Medinipur, West Bengal.
Dr. Brijesh Chandra Yadav, Anaesthesia Resident, Motilal Nehru Medical College, Allahabad.
Dr. Sumi Maniraju, MBBS, Vinayaka Mission's Medical College and Hospital, Karaikal.
Dr. Vennila Krishnan, MBBS, Sri Muthukumaran Medical College and Hospital, Chennai.
Dr. Shanmugasundaram, MBBS, IGMC and RI, Puducherry.
Dr. Ramayee, MBBS, Junior Resident in OBG, IGMC and RI, Puducherry.
Dr. Kalaivani, MBBS, Junior Resident in OBG, IGMC and RI, Puducherry.
Dr. Zubaida Begum A, MBBS (MGMC and RI), Junior Resident in Department of PSM, IGMC and RI, Puducherry.
Dr. Priyadharshini A, MBBS (SVMCH and RC), MRB, Tamil Nadu.
Dr. Maheswaran, MBBS, Government Stanley Medical College, Chennai.
Dr. Vishnu Venkatesan, MBBS SVMCHRC, Puducherry.
Dr. Supriya Jeevanthanam, MBBS, Government Vellore Medical College, Vellore.
Dr. Rachit Singhania, MBBS, North Bengal Medical College and Hospital, Darjeeling, West Bengal.
Dr. Renuga Devi, MBBS, Junior Resident in Pediatrics, MAPIMS, Melmaruvathur, Tamil Nadu.
Dr. Shahul Hamid, MBBS, IGMC and RI, Puducherry.
Dr. Ashwin Reddy, MBBS, IGMC and RI, Puducherry.
Dr. Jayaram Saibaba, MBBS, Medicine Junior Resident, JIPMER, Puducherry.
Dr. Immaneul Joshua, MBBS, IGMC and RI, Puducherry.
Dr. GK Raman, MBBS, IGMC and RI, Puducherry.
Dr. Ashok E, MBBS, DCH, Salem, Tamil Nadu.
Dr. Anandhasayanan Sriramalu, MBBS, Tirukkoyilur, Tamil Nadu

and

Mr. Thirunavukkarasu D, Government School English Lecturer (Retd), Puducherry.
Mrs. Sampurnam, Principal (Retd), SSVHSS, Puducherry.
Mr. Vijayan D, Cash Officer (Retd), SBI, Puducherry.
Mrs. Sagoundala, Under Secretary (Retd), Government of Puducherry.
Mr. Srinivasan@Babu, PWD, Puducherry.
Mr. Dhinesh Shankar, EC Software, Chennai.
Mr. Rajkumar, System Engineer, Apple, CA, USA.

Write to Us

Any observations, suggestions, criticisms are welcome. Write to the author at babuarun.t@gmail.com

Errata

Please visit www.drarunbabu.in and www.peepeepub.com

Follow Author in Facebook: www.facebook.com/targetjipmer/ and Dr Arun Babu's Pediatrics Discussion group (TARGET Pediatrics by Dr Arun Babu)

CONTENTS

JIPMER–MAY 2019

ANATOMY

1. When does the marked structure (Black arrow) close in utero?

(a) 30 days (b) 25 days
(c) 12 days (d) 7 days

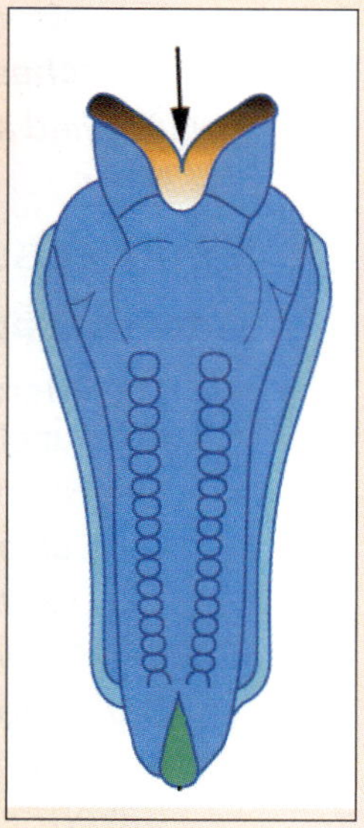

Explanation:

- Picture is showing dorsal view of neural tube at approximately **23 days***. Black arrow indicates the **anterior neuropore***.

Neural Tube Development

- **Neuropores** are the openings in the cranial and caudal ends of neural tube.
  - ***Cranial neuropore*** (**anterior**) closes at approximately ***day 25*** [18-20 somite stage]
  - ***Caudal neuropore*** (**posterior**) closes at ***day 28*** [25 somite stage]
- Neural tube develops from **neuroectoderm** and gives rise to **brain** and **spinal cord.**
  - *Failure of closure of **anterior neuropore** leads to **anencephaly****
  - *Failure of closure of **posterior neuropore** leads to **spina bifida*** (**lumbosacral region**)
- Neural tube defects can be ***prevented by*** administration of ***400 μg of folic acid daily*** beginning 3 months prior to conception and continuing throughout pregnancy.
- When ***Family history of present or history of previous child with neural tube defects*** it is recommended that she must take ***400 μg of folic acid daily and then 4,000 μg per day starting 1 month before she tries to become pregnant*** and continuing through first trimester.

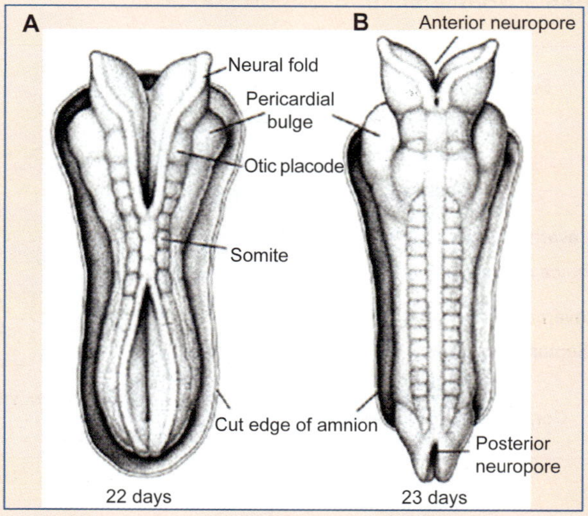

Figure: Dorsal view of Neural tubes on 22 days and 23 days

Ans: (b) 25 days

Ref: *Langman's Medical Embryology, TW Sadler, 13th edition, 2015, Page 73 and 74*

2. Dorsal artery of penis passes beneath which layer?

(a) Colle's fascia
(b) Buck's fascia
(c) Dartos layer
(d) Tunica albuginea

Explanation:

Dorsal artery of the penis

- The dorsal artery of the penis is a *branch from* ***common penile artery**** which is a branch from **internal pudendal artery*.**
- Dorsal artery of the penis runs alongside the **dorsal vein** and the **dorsal penile nerve**, and is attached, together with these structures, to the ***underside of Buck's fascia*.***
- ***Branches***–It gives off **circumferential branches** to the **corpus spongiosum*** and **urethra*** .
- ***Applied anatomy***–Rich blood supply to the spongiosum allows safe division of the urethra during stricture repair.

EXTRA EDGE:

Arteries supplying penis:

- The **internal pudendal artery**, a branch of the **internal iliac artery**, gives off the ***common penile artery*** that supplies the **deep structures** of the penis.
- The common penile artery has ***three main branches***:
  - *Bulbourethral artery (artery to the bulb)*
  - *Dorsal penile artery*
  - *Cavernous (deep artery) artery*
- ***Bulbourethral artery***–Penetrates the perineal membrane to enter the spongiosum and supplies the **penile bulb** and the **urethra**, in addition to the **corpus spongiosum** and **glans penis**.
- ***Cavernous or deep artery of the penis***–Usually a paired vessel that ***pierces the tunica albuginea*** of the corpora cavernosa at the hilum of the penis and then travels near the centre of the corporal bodies in the direction of the glans penis.

Fascia covering the penis:

- The ***superficial penile fascia (Colle's fascia)*** consists of loose connective tissue interspersed by fibers of the **dartos muscle** from the **scrotum**; it is commonly referred to as the **dartos layer**.
- The ***deep penile fascia*** is a denser fascial sheath, known as ***Buck's fascia***, which envelops both **corpora cavernosa** and splits to envelop the **corpus spongiosum.**
- The ***tunica albuginea*** covering all three corporal bodies.

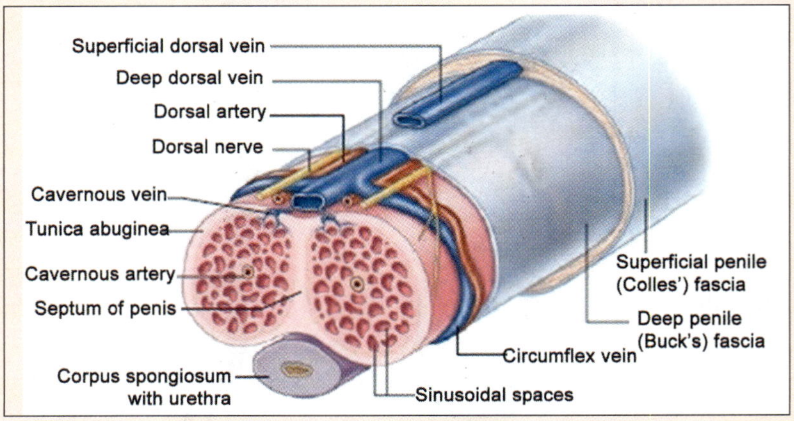

Figure: Layers of the penis and main structures

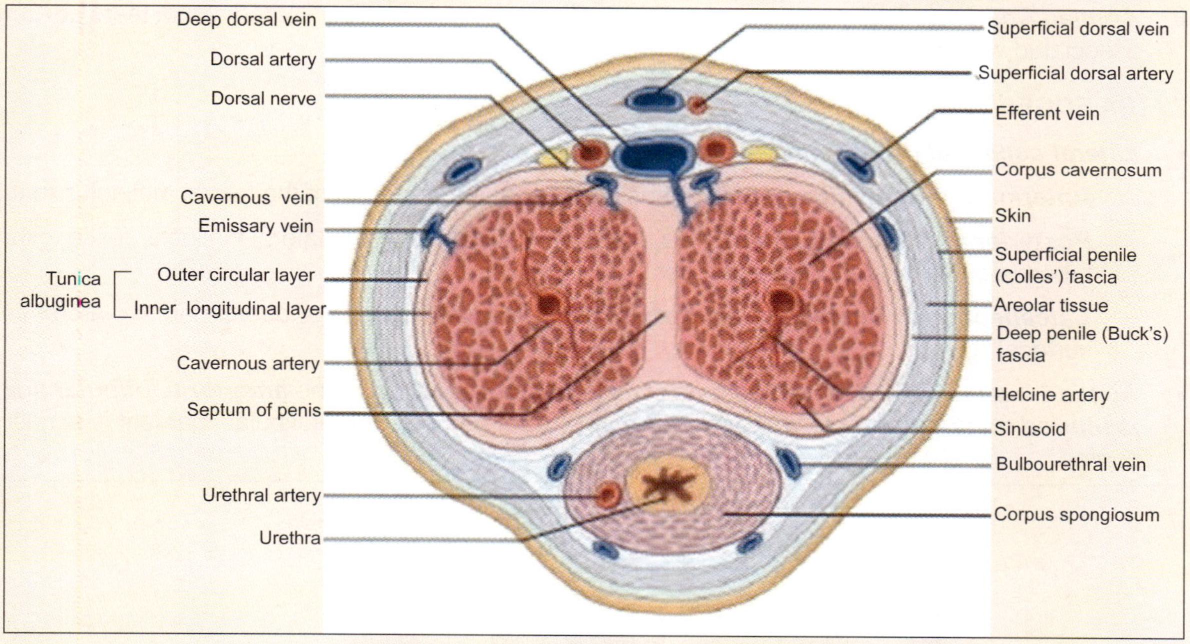

Figure: Cross-sectional anatomy of the penile shaft

Ans: (b) Buck's fascia

Ref: *Gray's Anatomy, The Anatomical Basis of Clinical Practice, Susan Standring, 41st edition, 2015, Page 1283 and 1284*

3. Deltoid ligament contains which of the following?

(a) Tibiotalar ligament
(b) Talofibular ligament
(c) Talonavicular ligament
(d) Calceneocuboid

Explanation:

Deltoid ligament/Medial collateral ligament

- **Medial collateral ligament*** of **ankle joint** also called **deltoid ligament***
- It is a strong, triangular band, attached to the medial malleolus
- This ligament has ***superficial and deep part***
  1. ***Superficial part*** has ***3 sets of fibers – Anterior, intermediate and posterior fibers***
     (a) ***Anterior fibers*** also called ***tibionavicular fibers*** [pass anteriorly to the navicular tuberosity]
     (b) ***Intermediate fibers*** also called ***tibiocalcaneal fibers*** [descend almost vertically to the entire length of the sustentaculum tali of calcaneum]
     (c) ***Posterior fibers*** also called ***superficial posterior tibiotalar fibers*** [pass posterolaterally to the medial side of the talus and its medial tubercle]
  2. ***Deep part*** also has 3 set of fibers–***anterior, intermediate and posterior fibers***
     (a) ***Anterior tibiotalar fibers*** [pass from the medial malleolus to the non-articular part of the medial talar surface]
     (b) ***Intermediate fibers*** deep to the tibiocalcaneal ligament [descend almost vertically to the entire length of the sustentaculum tali]
     (c) ***Posterior fibers (deep posterior tibiotalar)*** [pass posterolaterally to the medial side of the talus and its medial tubercle]

- ***Applied Anatomy:*** The medial collateral ligament of the ankle is rarely injured alone: tears are commonly associated with **a fracture of the distal fibula***.

EXTRA EDGE:

- ***Lateral collateral ligament of ankle*** has three discrete parts:
  - ***Anterior talofibular ligament*** [extends from the anterior margin of the lateral malleolus to the talus]
  - ***Posterior talofibular ligament*** [runs almost horizontally from the lateral malleolar fossa to the lateral tubercle of the posterior talar process]
  - ***Calcaneofibular ligament*** [from apex of the lateral malleolus to a tubercle on the lateral calcaneal surface]
- ***Applied Anatomy:*** The lateral ligament complex – more specifically, the ***anterior talofibular ligament – is injured most commonly with inversion sprains****; the posterior talofibular ligament is almost always spared.

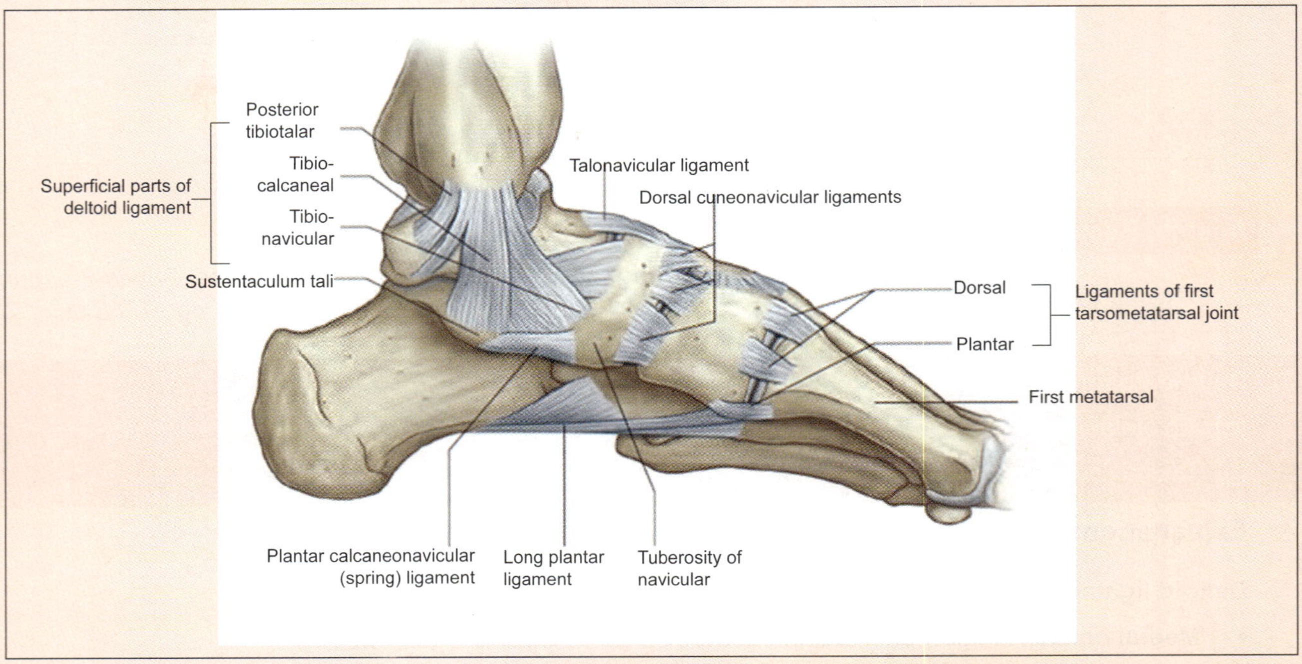

Figure: The left ankle and tarsal joints – medial aspect

Ans: (a) Tibiotalar ligament

Ref: *Gray's Anatomy, The Anatomical Basis of Clinical Practice, Susan Standring, 41st edition, 2015, Page 1431*

4. True statement regarding Kugel's anastomotic artery is:

(a) Arising directly from arch of aorta
(b) From left anterior descending coronary artery
(c) From left circumflex artery
(d) Artery connected to coronary sinus

Explanation:

Kugel's anastomotic artery

- Also called **arteria anastomotica auricularis magna***
- Present in **6%** of population
- Anastomotic communication between branches of the **proximal left circumflex artery*** with the **distal right coronary artery***.

- An **atrial branch** of **circumflex artery** [branch from **left coronary artery**] anastomoses with **similar branch** of **right coronary artery** along the **anterior atrial wall.**

Origin

- **Left circumflex artery (LCx)**
    - Most common variant proximal LCx to distal right coronary artery
    - Less commonly will end in the distal LCx
- **Right coronary artery (RCA)**
    - Most commonly terminating in a more distal segment of right coronary artery
    - May also communicate with the left circumflex artery via the sinoatrial nodal artery

Ans: (c) From left circumflex artery

Ref: *Gray's Anatomy, The Anatomical Basis of Clinical Practice, Susan Standring, 41st edition, 2015, Page 1020*

5. A sportsperson presents with laceration of wrist but with no vascular injury. On examination, a structure lateral to flexor digitorum superficialis is found to be injured. What action he most likely cannot perform?

(a) Opposition of thumb
(b) Adduction of 2nd digit
(c) Abduction of 2nd digit
(d) Flexion of thumb

Explanation:

- Structure present lateral to the flexor digitorum superficialis at the level of wrist is ***flexor pollicis longus****
- ***Flexor pollicis longus:*** Originates from the anterior surface of the **radius** and the adjacent half of the anterior surface of the **interosseous membrane**
- Its tendon passes through the carpal tunnel, ***lateral to the tendons of flexor digitorum superficialis and flexor digitorum profundus muscles***
- It is inserted into the **base of the distal phalanx of thumb**
- ***Action:*** **Flexes** the **thumb** at **MCP and IP** joints
- ***Nerve supply:*** **Anterior interosseous nerve** (branch of the **median nerve**)

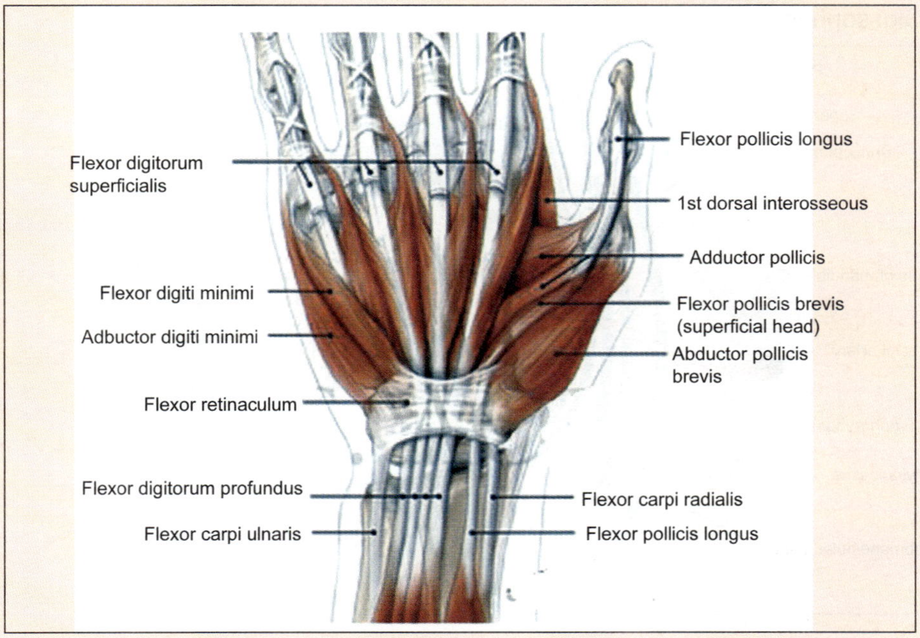

Ans: (d) Flexion of thumb

Ref: *Gray's Anatomy for Students, Richard L Drake,WayneVogl and Adam W.M.Mitchell, 2007, Page 697 and 698*

6. During tonsillectomy, which of the following structure is not injured?

(a) Tonsillar branch of facial artery
(b) External carotid artery
(c) Glossopharyngeal nerve
(d) Paratonsillar vein

Explanation:

- During tonsillectomy, because of the rich blood supply of the tonsil bleeding commonly arises from the large ***external palatine vein (paratonsillar vein)*** or, less commonly, from the ***tonsillar artery or other arterialtwigs***.
- The ***glossopharyngeal nerve*** accompanies the tonsillar artery on the lateral wall of the pharynx. Because this wall is thin, the nerve is vulnerable to injury.
- The ***internal carotid artery*** is especially vulnerable when it is tortuous and lies directly lateral to the tonsil.

Structures forming/related to the tonsillar bed:

- ***Muscles and fascia:***
  - Pharyngobasillar fascia
  - Palatopharyngeus muscle
  - Superior constrictor muscle
  - Styloglossus muscle
- ***Arteries:***
  - Facial artery and its ascending palatine branch
  - Ascending pharyngeal artery
  - Internal carotid artery (lies about 25 mm behind and lateral to the tonsil)
- ***Vein:***
  - Paratonsillar vein
- ***Nerve:***
  - Glossopharyngeal nerve

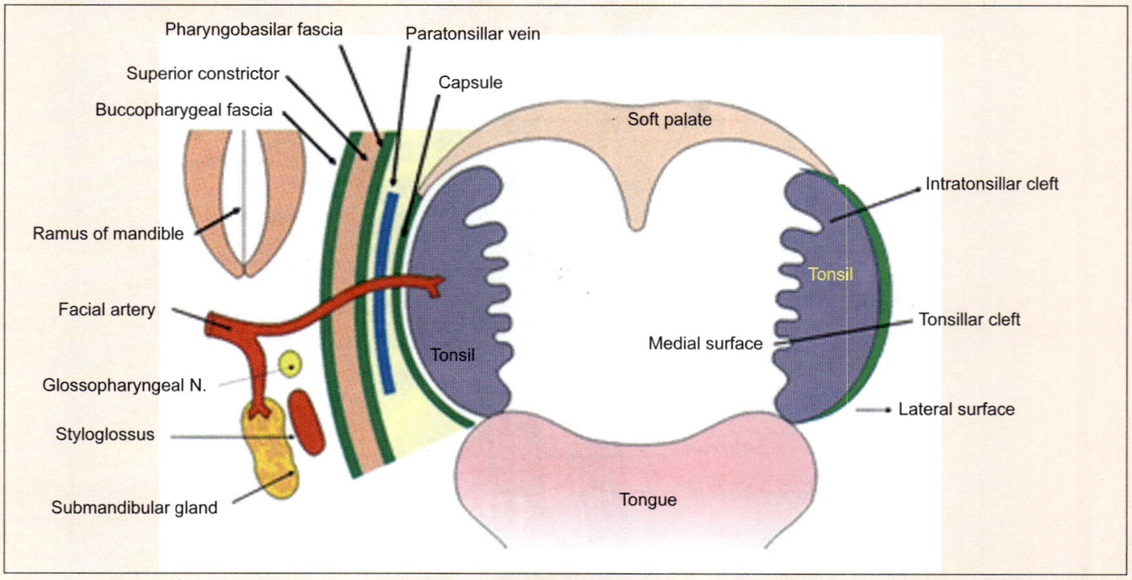

Figure: Structures forming/related to the tonsillar bed

Ans: (b) External carotid artery

Ref: *Moore Clinically Oriented Anatomy, Keith L. Moore, Arthur F Dalley and Anne M R Agur, 7th edition, 2014, Page 1035 and 1047*

7. Which structure is not passing through the gap between superior and middle constrictor muscle of pharynx?

(a) Glossopharyngeal nerve
(b) Stylopharyngeus muscle
(c) Internal laryngeal nerve
(d) Both stylopharyngeus and Glossopharyngeal nerves

Explanation:

- Structures passing through the gap between **superior and middle constrictor** muscle are **Stylopharyngeus muscle and Glossopharyngeal nerve***

Gap in the pharynx	Structures passing through	
Gap between the **base of Skull and upper border of Superior constrictor [Sinus of Morgagni*]**	• Auditory tube • Tensor velipalatini • Levator veli palatini • Ascending palatine artery	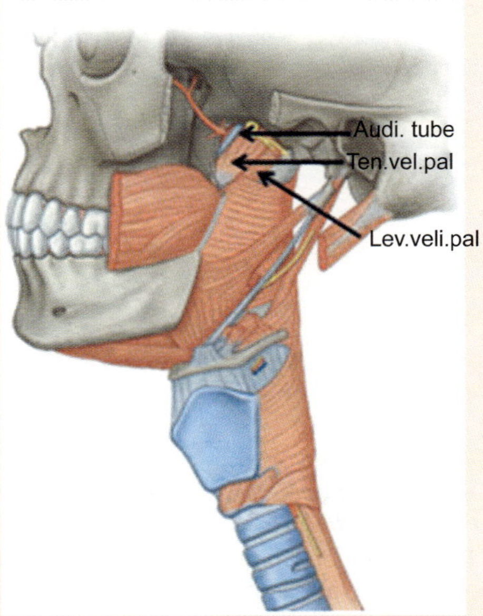
Gap between **Superior constrictor and Middle constrictor**	• Stylopharyngeus muscle* • Glossopharyngeal nerve*	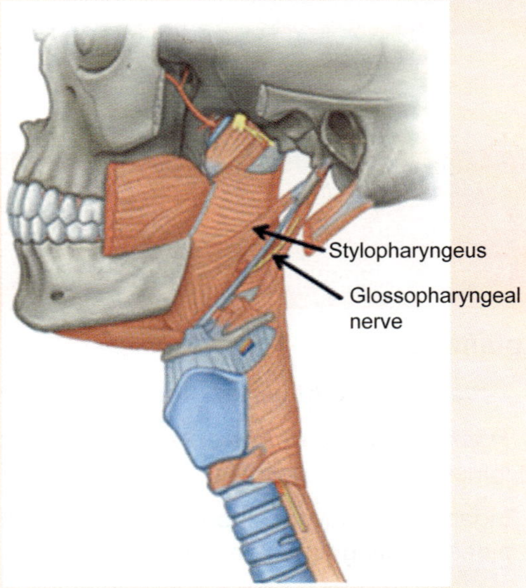

Contd.

Contd.

Gap between **Middle constrictor and Inferior constrictor**	• Internal laryngeal nerve • Superior laryngeal vessels	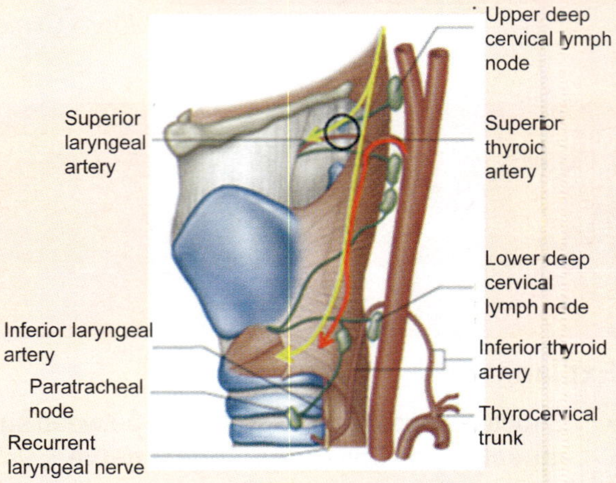
Gap between **Inferior constrictor and oesophagus**	• Recurrent laryngeal nerve* • Inferior laryngeal vessels*	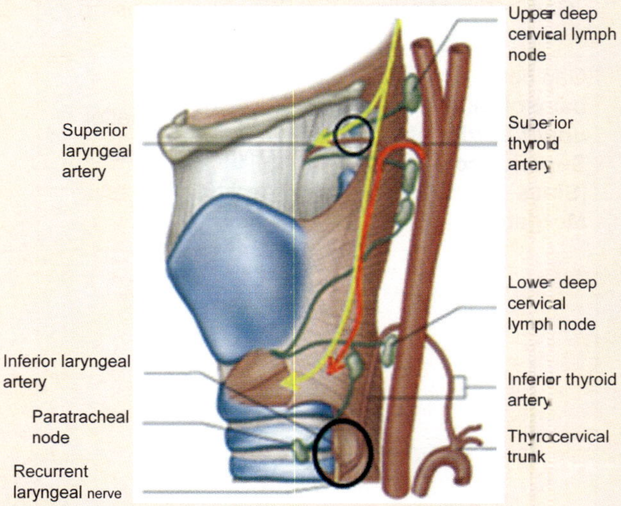

- ***Hypopharyngeal diverticula*** occur in the lower portion of the pharynx through areas of weakness in the pharyngeal wall.
- The pharyngeal mucosa that lies between **cricopharyngeus** and **thyropharyngeus** is relatively unsupported by pharyngeal muscles and is called the ***Killian's dehiscence.***

Ans: (c) Internal laryngeal nerve

Ref: *Gray's Anatomy for Students, Richard L Drake, WayneVogl and Adam W.M.Mitchell, 2007, Page 942 and 943*

8. Structure forming the posterior 1/3rd of vertebral canal is:

(a) Posterior 1/3rd of vertebral body
(b) Posterior 1/3rd of intervertebral disc
(c) Posterior longitudinal ligament
(d) Ligamentum flavum

Explanation:

- ***Anterior 2/3rd of vertebral canal*** is formed by **vertebral body** and **intervertebral disc** (posterior part).
- ***Posterior 1/3rd of vertebral canal*** is formed by the **laminae of adjacent vertebral arches**, which are joined by broad, pale yellow bands of elastic tissue called the ***ligamentum flavum***.
- Ligamentum flavum extends almost vertically from the lamina above to the lamina below, those of opposite sides meeting and blending in the midline.

- The ***flaval ligaments*** bind the lamina of the adjoining vertebrae together, forming alternating sections of the ***posterior wall of the vertebral canal***.
- The ligament flava are long, thin and broad in the cervical region, thicker in the thoracic region, and thickest in the lumbar region.
- Flaval ligaments resist separation of the vertebral lamina by limiting abrupt flexion of the vertebral column, and thereby prevent injury to the IV discs.
- The strong, elastic yellow ligaments help preserve the normal curvatures of the vertebral column and assist with straightening of the column after flexing.
- ***Posterior longitudinal ligament*** forms the **anterior wall** of **vertebral canal.**
- ***Anterior longitudinal ligament*** lines the **anterior surface** of **vertebral body.**

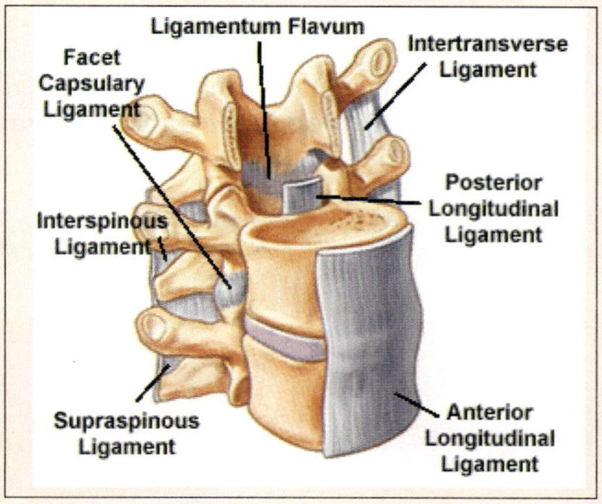

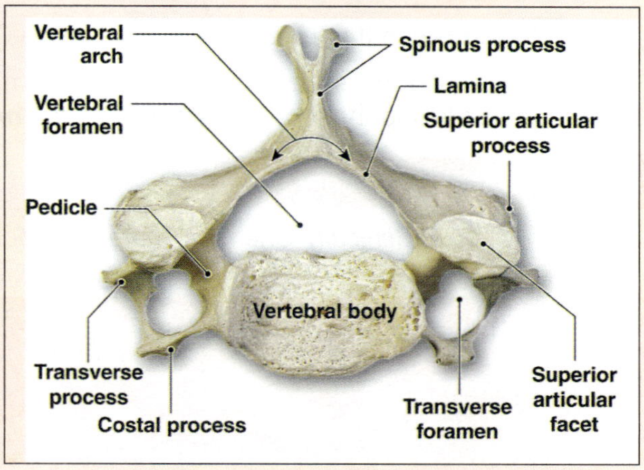

ALSO NOTE:

Contents of Vertebral Canal

- Spinal meninges
- Spinal cord with its nerve roots and vessels
- Epidural space (extradural space) containing
  - Loose connective tissue
  - Fat
  - Veins (Internal vertebral venous plexus)

Ans: (d) Ligamentum flavum

Ref: *Moore Clinically Oriented Anatomy, Keith L Moore, Arthur F Dalley and Anne M R and Agur, 7th edition, 2014, Page 466*

9. While doing excision of cervical lymph nodes, inadvertent injury to which nerve causes drooping of shoulder?

(a) Suprascapular nerve
(b) Spinal accessory nerve
(c) Supraclavicular nerve
(d) Nerve to serratus anterior

Explanation:

Spinal Accessory Nerve (CN XI):

- Supplies **sternocleidomastoid** and **trapezius** muscles (elevation of scapula/shrugging of shoulder)

Lesions of Spinal Accessory Nerve (CN XI):

- **Drooping of the shoulder** is an obvious sign of **CN XI injury**.
- **Unilateral paralysis** of the trapezius is evident by the patient's **inability** to **elevate** and **retract** the **shoulder** and by difficulty in elevating the upper limb superior to the horizontal level.
- Lesions of the spinal accessory nerve (CN XI) are uncommon.
- This nerve may be damaged by:
  - Penetrating trauma, such as a stab or bullet wound.
  - During extensive ***surgical dissections in the lateral cervical region***—for example, during removal of cancerous lymph nodes—the surgeon isolates CN XI to preserve it, if possible.
  - Tumors at the cranial base or ***cancerous cervical lymph nodes***.
  - **Fractures** of the **jugular foramen**, where CN XI leaves the cranium.
  - Awareness of superficial location of this nerve during superficial procedures in the lateral cervical region is important because ***CN XI is the most commonly involved in iatrogenic nerve injury.***

Ans: (b) Spinal accessory nerve

Ref: *Clinically Oriented Anatomy, Moore Keith L, Dalley, Arthur F, 5th Edition, 2006, Page 1061*

10. All are Neural crest derivatives except:

(a) Sympathetic ganglia
(b) Muscles of ciliary body
(c) C cells of thyroid gland
(d) Odontoblasts

Explanation:

Neural crest derivatives

- Connective tissue and bones of the face and skull
- Cranial nerve ganglia
- **"C" cells of the thyroid gland***
- **Conotruncal septum** in the heart
- **Odontoblasts***
- Dermis in face and neck
- Spinal (dorsal root) ganglia
- Sympathetic chain and preaortic ganglia
- Parasympathetic ganglia of the gastrointestinal tract
- **Adrenal medulla***
- **Schwann cells***
- Glial cells
- Meninges
- **Melanocytes***
- **Smooth muscle cells to blood vessels of the face and forebrain***

Note:

- **Sphincter pupillae** and **dilator pupillae muscles** develop from **neuroectoderm** of optic cup.
- ***Ciliary muscles*** developed from ***mesenchyme*** [mesenchyme occupying the region between the optic cup and the overlying surface epithelium].

EXTRA EDGE:

Optic Cup Derivatives:

- Optic cup has ***outer and inner layers***:
    - ***Outer layer*** is known as the ***pigmented layer of the retina*** [characterized by small pigment granules]
- ***Inner layer*** [neural layer]
    - The ***posterior four-fifths*** of inner layer–***pars optica retinae*** [differentiate into retina]
    - The ***anterior one-fifth*** of the inner layer–***pars ceca retinae***
    - It divides into the ***pars iridica retinae*** [forms the inner layer of the iris] and the ***pars ciliaris retinae*** [forms the ciliary body]
- The region between the optic cup and the overlying surface epithelium is filled with loose mesenchyme.
- The ***sphincter and dilator pupillae*** muscles forms within this tissue and these muscles are migrated and developed from the underlying neuroectoderm of the optic cup.
- The ***pars ciliaris retinae*** is externally covered by a layer of mesenchyme that forms the ***ciliary muscle*** and on the innerside it is connected to the lens by a network of elastic fibers, the ***suspensory ligament or zonula.***

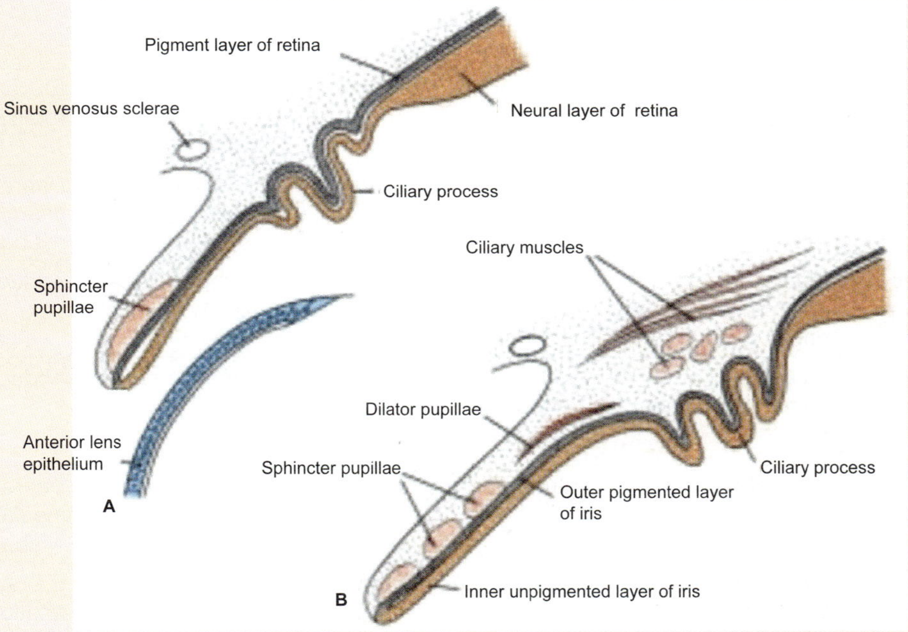

Development of the iris and ciliary body. The rim of the optic cup is covered by mesenchyme, in which the sphincter and dilator pupillae develop from the underlying

Ans: (b) Muscles of ciliary body

Ref: *Langman's Medical Embryology, TW Sadler, 13th edition, 2015, Page 77*

11. True about superior oblique origin and insertion:

(a) Originate from lesser wing of sphenoid and inserted into sclera in front of equator

(b) Originate from common tendinous ring (ring of Zinn) and inserted into sclera behind the equator

(c) Originate from greater wing of sphenoid and inserted into sclera in front of equator

(d) Originate from the body of sphenoid and inserted into the sclera behind the equator

Explanation:

Superior oblique muscle:

- ***Origin:*** Superior oblique muscle that arises from the ***body of the sphenoid*** superomedial to the optic canal and the tendinous attachment of the superior rectus.
- ***Course:*** It runs forward to end in around tendon that passes through a fibrocartilaginous loop [trochlea] attached to the trochlear fossa of the frontal bone.
- ***Insertion:*** The tendon subsequently descends posterolaterally and inferior to superior rectus, and is attached to the ***sclera*** in the superolateral part of ***the posterior quadrant behind the equator***, between the superior and lateral recti.
- ***Vascular supply:*** **Ophthalmic artery** and its **supraorbital branch.**
- ***Nerve supply:*** **Trochlear nerve*.**
- ***Actions:*** **Depression, abduction and intorsion.**

Extra-ocular muscles:

Muscle	Origin	Insertion	Nerve supply	Actions
Levator palpebrae superioris	Lesser wing of sphenoid anterior to optic canal	Anterior surface of tarsal plate; a few fibers to skin and superior conjunctival fornix	**Oculomotor nerve** [III]–superior branch	**Elevation** of upper eyelid
Superior rectus	Superior part of common tendinous ring (ring of Zinn)	Anterior half of eyeball superiorly	Oculomotor nerve [III]–superior branch	Elevation, adduction, medial rotation (intorsion) of eyeball
Inferior rectus	Inferior part of common tendinous ring	Anterior half of eyeball inferiorly	Oculomotor nerve [III]–inferior branch	Depression, adduction, lateral rotation (extorsion) of eyeball
Medial rectus	Medial part of common tendinous ring	Anterior half of eyeball medially	Oculomotor nerve [III]–inferior branch	Adduction of eyeball
Lateral rectus	Lateral part of common tendinous ring	Anterior half of eyeball laterally	**Abducent nerve** [VI]*	Abduction of eyeball
Superior oblique	Body of sphenoid, superior and medial to optic canal	Outer posterior quadrant of eyeball	**Trochlear nerve** [IV]*	Depression, abduction, medial rotation (intorsion) of eyeball
Inferior oblique	Medial floor of orbit posterior to rim; maxilla lateral to nasolacrimal groove	Outer posterior quadrant of eyeball	Oculomotor nerve [III]–inferior branch	Elevation, abduction, lateral rotation (extorsion) of eyeball

Ans: (d) Originate from the body of sphenoid and inserted into the sclera behind the equator

Ref: *Gray's Anatomy, The Anatomical Basis of Clinical Practice, Susan Standring, 41st Edition, 2015, Page 671 and Gray's Anatomy for Students, Richard L Drake, Wayne Vogl and Adam WM Mitchell, 2007, Page 840*

12. Persistence of omphalomesenteric duct is:

(a) Gastroschisis (b) Omphalocele
(c) Meckel's diverticulum (d) Ectopia vesicae

Explanation:

Meckel's diverticulum or ileal diverticulum:

- It is the ***persistent proximal part of omphalomesenteric duct or vitellointestinal duct.***

- It is a ***true diverticulum*** that includes all the 4 layers of intestine.
- Present in ***2 to 4%*** of people.
- A small portion of the vitelline duct persists, forming an outpocketing of the ileum.
- Approximately **40 to 60 cm** [***approximately 2 feet***] from the ileocecal valve on the ***antimesenteric border*** of the ileum.
- Does not usually cause any symptoms. However, when it contains ***heterotopic pancreatic tissue or gastric mucosa***, it may cause ***ulceration, bleeding, or even perforation.***
- ***Enterocystoma or vitelline cyst***–sometimes both ends of the vitelline duct transform into fibrous cords, and the middle portion forms a large cyst.
- Since the fibrous cords traverse the peritoneal cavity, intestinal loops may twist around the fibrous strands and become obstructed, causing ***strangulation or volvulus.***
- ***Umbilical fistula, or vitelline fistula***–vitelline duct remains patent over its entire length forming a direct communication between the umbilicus and the intestinal tract. A fecal discharge may then be found at the umbilicus.

Ans: (c) Meckel's diverticulum

Ref: *Langman's Medical Embryology, TW Sadler,13th edition, 2016, Page 311 and 312*

13. Which of the following is a derivative of second arch?

(a) Malleus (b) Stapes

(c) Maxilla (d) Mandible

Explanation:

Pharyngeal arches and their derivatives

Arch number	Arch name	Embryonic cartilage	Cartilage derivative	Muscle	Nerve	Artery
1	**Mandibular**	Quadrate Meckel's	• Incus* • Malleus* • Anterior ligament of malleus • Spine of sphenoid • Sphenomandibular ligament • Genial tubercle of mandible	• Tensor tympani • Muscles of mastication • Mylohyoid • Anterior belly of digastric • Tensor veli palatini	**Trigeminal (V) Mandibular division**	• First aortic arch artery [transitory]
2	**Hyoid**	Reichert's	• **Stapes*** • Styloid process of temporal bone • Stylohyoid ligament • Lesser horn and upper part of Body of hyoid bone	• Stapedius • Stylohyoid • Facial muscles, including: – Buccinator – Platysma – Posterior belly of digastric	**Facial** (VII)	• Stapedial artery [transitory]
3	Third		• Greater horn and lower part of body of hyoid	• Stylopharyngeus	**Glosso-pharyngeal** (IX)	• Common carotid artery, first part of internal carotid artery

Contd.

Contd.

4	Fourth		• Thyroid cartilage • Corniculate cartilage • Cunieform cartilage	• Pharyngeal and extrinsic laryngeal muscles, levator veli palatini	**Vagus** (X) **Pharyngeal** branch	• Proximal part of subclavian artery on the right side • Arch of aorta between origins of left common carotid and left subclavian arteries
6	Sixth		• Arytenoid cartilages	• Intrinsic laryngeal muscles	**Vagus** (X) recurrent **laryngeal** branch	• Part between the pulmonary trunk and dorsal aorta • Becomes **ductus arteriosus on left**, disappears on right

Ans: (b) Stapes

Ref: *Gray's Anatomy, 40th edition, Page 596*

14. Crystalline Lens is derived from:

(a) Surface ectoderm (b) Neuroectoderm
(c) Mesoderm (d) Endoderm

Explanation:

Embryology of Eye

- The developing eye appears in the **22 days** embryo as a pair of shallow grooves on the sides of the forebrain.
- Optic vesicle forms as an out pocketings of the forebrain which comes in contact with the **surface ectoderm.**
- The optic vesicle begin to invaginate to form **optic cup.**
- The cells of surface ectoderm initially in contact with the optic vesicle begin to elongate and form the lens placode which develops into lens **vesicle.**
- The lens develops from the lens vesicle.
- The posterior cells become filled with a very high concentration of proteins (**crystallins**) which **render them transparent**; they also become densely packed within the lens as **primary lens fibers**.

- Cells at the equatorial region of the lens elongate and contribute secondary lens fibers to the body of the lens in a process which continues into adult life.
- The polarity and growth of the lens appear to depend on the differential distribution of soluble factors which promote either cell division or lens fiber differentiation and are present in the anterior chamber and vitreous humour respectively.
- Congenital cataracts can be associated with mutations in genes that encode structural lens proteins, particularly **crystallin proteins**.

Embryogenic orgin of Eye structures

Surface Ectoderm	Neural Ectoderm	Mesoderm	Neural Crest
• Conjunctival epithelium • Corneal epithelium • ***Crystalline lens*** • Tarsal glands • Lacrimal glands	• Iris epithelium • Ciliary epithelium • ***Sphincter pupillae*** • ***Dilator pupillae*** • Part of vitreous • Part of retina • Part of RPE • Part of optic nerve	• ***Extraocular muscle*** • Corneal stroma • ***Sclera*** • Iris stroma • ***Choroid*** • Vessels • Part of vitreous	• Corneal endothelium • Trabecular meshwork endothelium • ***Ciliary muscle*** • Part of vitreous • Uveal melanocytes • Meningeal sheaths of optic nerve • Ciliary ganglion

Ans: (a) Surface ectoderm

Ref: *Gray's Anatomy, 40th edition, Page 700*

PHYSIOLOGY

1. Incretins cause:

(a) Decrease in insulin secretion
(b) Increase in blood glucose levels
(c) Increase in glucagon levels
(d) Increase in insulin secretion

Explanation:

Incretins

- Incretins are the gastrointestinal hormones secreted by **enteroendocrine cells** which sense the nutrients in the GI tract, especially **glucose**.
- **Gastric Inhibitory Peptide (GIP)** and **Glucagon like peptide-1 (GLP-1)** are the two incretins found in humans. They increase the ability of blood glucose to stimulate insulin secretion from the β cells of pancreas.
- GIP also known as **glucose-dependent insulinotropic peptide,** is secreted by **K cells** of **small intestines**.
- GLP-1 is secreted by the **L cells of intestine**. In addition to its insulin stimulatory effect, **GLP-1 suppresses glucagon secretion***, **delays gastric emptying***, and **reduces apoptosis** of human **islets*** in culture.
- GIP and GLP-1 act through **Gs-coupled receptors** on cells, which increase **cAMP**.
- Incretins also enhances the synthesis of **glucose transporter**, **GLUT-2 and hexokinase**.
- The ability of incretins to increase insulin secretion is strongly dependent on circulating glucose levels. The effect of incretins is terminated once the blood glucose levels fall. Hence, there is low risk of development of severe hypoglycemia with incretin analogs.
- GLP-1 receptor agonists such as **exenatide, liraglutide, albiglutide, and dulaglutide** are available for treating Type II Diabetes Mellitus.

Factors affecting insulin secretion

- Other intestinal hormones that stimulate insulin secretion include **gastrin**, **secretin** and **Cholecystokinin***.
- Major stimuli for insulin secretion include **increased serum glucose** and **certain amino acids such as leucine and arginine.**
- **Cholinergic (muscarinic) receptor activation** also increases insulin secretion, whereas **α2-adrenergic receptors** inhibit insulin secretion.

Ans: (d) Increase in insulin secretion

Ref: *Bruce White, Endocrine and Reproductive Physiology, 4th edition, Page 38, Ganong's Review of Medical Physiology, 26th edition; Bertram G Katzung Basic and Clinical Pharmacology, 14th edition, Page 761*

2. A man weighing 60 kg has 45% hematocrit. What will be his plasma volume?

(a) 2640
(b) 3080
(c) 3850
(d) 3300

Explanation:

- Total blood volume constitutes both **plasma volume and blood cell volume**.
- Total blood volume is about **80 ml/kg of body weight** or 8% of total body weight.

$$\text{Plasma Volume} = \text{Total Blood Volume} \times \frac{100 - \text{hematocrit}}{100}$$

In this question, Total blood volume can be calculated from body weight i.e.,

Assuming, Total blood volume as 80 ml/kg body weight

For 60 kg individual, total blood volume = 60 × 80 = 4800 mL.

$$\text{Hence, Plasma Volume} = 4800 \times \frac{100 - 45}{100} = 4800 \times 0.55 = 2640\text{ mL}$$

Measurement of body fluids

Compartment	Method
Total body water	**Deuterium oxide, Tritium oxide, antipyrine***
Extracellular fluid	Radioactive inulin, Mannitol, Sucrose, ^{25}Na, ^{125}I – iothalamate, thiosulfate
Intracellular fluid	TBW – ECF
Plasma volume	**Evan's blue dye**, ^{125}I albumin
Blood volume	BV = plasma volume/ (1- hematocrit), 51 Cr labelled RBCs
Interstitial fluid	ECF – Plasma volume

Ans: (a) 2640

Ref: *Ganong's Review of Medical Physiology, 26th edition, Page 4 and G.K.Pal Comprehensive Textbook of Medical Physiology, Page 63*

3. Respiratory parameter that does not change during pregnancy is:

(a) Inspiratory Reserve Volume (b) Tidal volume

(c) Respiratory rate (d) Expiratory reserve volume

Explanation:

MATERNAL CHANGES DURING PREGNANCY

(A) **Respiratory changes**

- Increase in minute ventilation
- Increase in tidal volume
- No change in respiratory rate
- Decrease in residual volume
- Decrease in Expiratory Reserve Volume
- Decrease in Functional Residual Capacity
- Increase in Inspiratory Reserve Volume

(B) **Cardiovascular Changes**

- Increase in plasma volume and red cell mass
- Increase in cardiac output due to increase in stroke volume and heart rate
- Decrease in peripheral resistance
- Increase in SBP
- Fall in DBP

(C) **Renal Changes**

- Glycosuria
- Increase in renal blood flow and GFR

(D) **Gastrointestinal changes**
- Reflux esophagitis due to reflux of gastric secretions
- Decreased GI motility

(E) **Endocrine changes**
- Increase in prolactin secretion
- Decrease in FSH and LH secretion
- Decrease in GH secretion
- TSH secretion is normal

Ans: (c) Respiratory rate

Ref: *G.K.Pal Comprehensive Textbook of Medical Physiology, 1st edition, Page 63 and Bruce White, Endocrine and Reproductive Physiology, 4th edition, Page 257*

4. In cardiac action potential, phase 0 is due to:

(a) Na^+K^+ ATPase (b) Sodium influx
(c) Potassium influx (d) Calcium influx

Explanation:

- The resting membrane potential of cardiac muscle cell is **-90mV**.
- Stimulation of the cell produces a propagated action potential that initiates contraction.

Phases of cardiac action potential

Phase 0	Initial **rapid depolarization** and overshoot	**Sodium influx** due to opening of voltage gated Na^+ channels
Phase 1	Initial **rapid repolarization**	Closure of **Na^+ channels** and opening of outward transient rectifying potassium channels that causes transient **outflux of K^+ ions**
Phase 2	**Plateau phase**	**Calcium influx** due to slower but prolonged opening of voltage gated L type Ca^{2+} channels (Calcium influx)
Phase 3	**Late rapid repolarization**	**Closure** of the **Ca^{2+} channels** and a slow, **delayed increase of K^+ efflux** through various types of K^+ channels
Phase 4	**Resting membrane potential***	

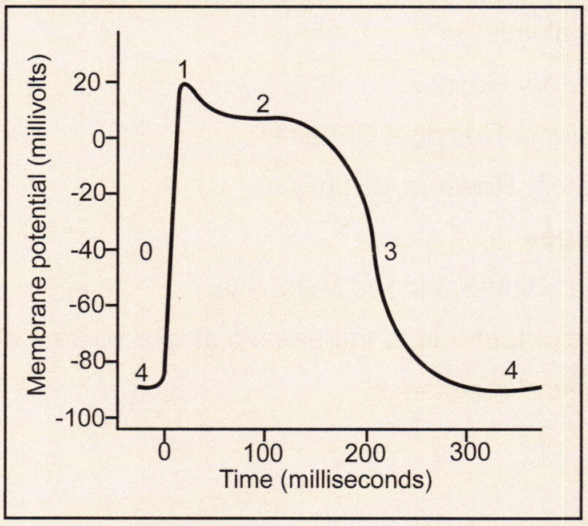

Figure: Cardiac action potential

Ans: (b) Sodium influx

Ref: *Ganong's Review of Medical Physiology, 26th edition, Page 520*

5. Calculate Oxygen Saturation Index with the following known parameters; FiO_2 – 0.6 PaO_2: 85 mm Hg; SpO_2: 90 and Mean Airway Pressure (MAP) – 12 cm H_2O:

(a) 8 (b) 8.5

(c) 7.5 (d) 10

Explanation:

Oxygen saturation index = [Mean Airway Pressure × FiO_2 × 100] ÷ SpO_2

= [12 × 0.6 × 100]/90= **8**

Oxygenation index and Oxygen saturation index

- **Oxygenation index = MAP× FiO_2**÷ PaO_2
  - FiO_2 = fraction of inhaled oxygen, %
  - MAP= mean airway pressure, cm of H_2O
  - PaO_2 = Partial pressure of arterial oxygen, mm Hg
- Oxygenation Index is considered to be a superior 'integrated' index of the **oxygenation efficiency** of the **lungs** during **mechanical ventilation** in Pediatric critical care. It is used to assess severity of **hypoxic respiratory failure** and **persistent pulmonary hypertension of the newborn**. Increase in Oxygenation index denotes worsening of the oxygenation status.
- Oxygenation index **more than 40*** signifies the need for **ECMO***.
- Measuring Oxygenation index is invasive and requires an indwelling arterial line or arterial puncture to obtain a blood gas sample. **Oxygen saturation index (OSI)** is less invasive procedure which helps as a surrogate to oxygenation index.

Ans: (a) 8

Ref: *Rawat M et al., Oxygen saturation index and severity of hypoxic respiratory failure, Neonatology 2015,107(3):161-6*

6. When an astronaut stays in microgravity for a prolonged period of time, which of the following occurs:

(a) Increase in bone mass (b) Increase in maximum cardiac output

(c) Increase red blood cell mass (d) Decrease in blood volume

Explanation:

- A person in an orbiting satellite experiences **weightlessness**, or a state of near-zero G force, which is also called **microgravity**.

Acute effects of microgravity:

- Blood volume redistributes towards the **head**. This cephalad shift of blood volume away from the capacitance vessels of the legs expands the central blood volume, increases the cardiac preload, and increases the filtration of plasma water into the interstitium of the facial region. This leads to **bloated facial appearance**.
- **Motion sickness** occurs for 2 to 5 days of stay in microgravity. This is due to altered inertial stimulation of the vestibular system in the absence of normal gravitational forces. It resolves within the first 96 hours of microgravity exposure as the vestibular system or the CNS accommodates to the novel input.

Effects of prolonged stay in space:

- Decrease in blood volume
- Impaired baroreceptor reflexes
- Reduced orthostatic tolerance
- Decrease in red blood cell mass

- Decrease in muscle strength and work capacity
- Decrease in maximum cardiac output
- Loss of calcium and phosphate from the bones leads to loss of bone mass

Ans: (d) Decrease in blood volume

Ref: *Guyton and Hall Textbook of Medical Physiology, 13th edition, Page 567 and Boron and Boulpaep, Medical Physiology, Updated edition, Page 1277*

7. Identify the cells marked in this picture:

(a) Ito cells (b) Hepatocyte

(c) Kupffer cells (d) Stellate cells

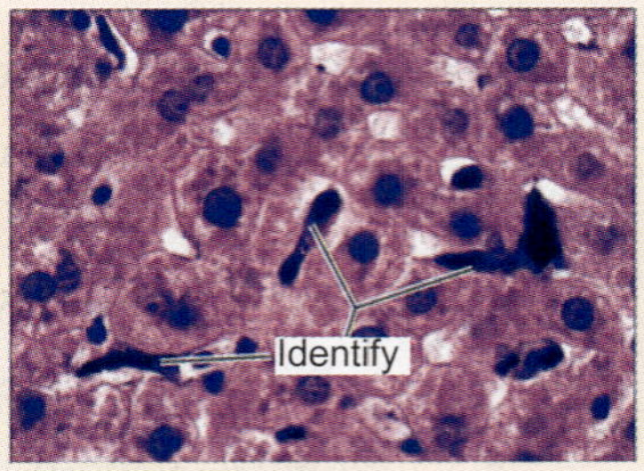

Explanation:

- HPE shows hepatic sinusoids with typical **Kupffer cells** (Arrows).

Kupffer cells (also known as stellate sinusoidal macrophages or Kupffer-Browicz cells)

- Specialized macrophages found in the **hepatic sinusoid**, along with sinusoidal endothelial cells, Ito cells and pit cells.
- Kupffer cells are **amoeboid-shaped** and are attached to the **sinusoidal endothelial cells**.
- Their surface contains **microvilli, pseudopodia and lamellipodia**, which can project out in all directions.
- The microvilli and pseudopodia are involved in **endocytosis** of particles.
- They also contain Golgi apparatus, ribosomes, centrioles, microfilaments, and microtubules in their cytoplasm.
- The nucleus is ovoid or indented and can be lobulated.
- They also contain rough endoplasmic reticulum, nuclear envelope, and annulate lamellae, which all contain **peroxidase activity.**
- Kupffer cells can be found in both the **centrilobular and periportal regions** in the liver, and their function and structures differ depending on their location.
- Kupffer cells in the
  - **In periportal regions** tend to be **larger**, have more **lysosomal enzyme activities**, and more **phagocytic activity.**
  - **In Centrilobular regions** produce **more superoxide anion.**
- The liver contains **endothelial cells, Kupffer cells and stellate cells (ito cells).**
- Kupffer cells are the **large phagocytic macrophages** that line the hepatic venous sinuses. They constitute about 15% of liver cells.
- German pathologist **Karl Von Kupffer** identified them using **gold impregnation technique**.
- Normally, Kupffer cells **break down senescent RBCs** via **phagocytosis** and **lysosomal degradation**. They remove **particulate matter** from the circulation.
- Hemosiderin, the iron containing pigment is stored in Kupffer cell which will be made available for new hemoglobin formation.
- Stellate cells are characterized by **large fat droplets** in the cytoplasm. They play a vital role in storage of **vitamin A**. On liver injury, stellate cells are activated and participate in **fibrogenesis** through remodeling of the extracellular matrix and deposition of type I collagen, which can lead to cirrhosis.

Ans: (c) Kupffer cells

Ref: *William K Ovalle, Netter's Essential Histology, 2nd edition, Page 321 and Boron and Boulpaep, Medical Physiology, Updated edition, Page 982*

8. Maximum forced expiration is primarily controlled by:

(a) Chest wall elasticity
(b) Diaphragm muscles
(c) Abdominal muscles
(d) Internal intercostal muscles

Explanation:

*"**Forced expiration** involves contraction of the **abdominal muscles** which forces the **diaphragm** upwards reducing the volume of the thoracic cavity. It also requires contraction of the **internal intercostal muscles** and **innermost intercostal muscles** which pull the ribs downwards." – Guyton*

Mechanics of pulmonary ventilation

- Expansion and contraction of lungs is accomplished by two ways:
  - Upward and downward movement of the diaphragm.
  - Increase and decrease in anteroposterior diameter of the chest wall.

Upward and downward movement of the diaphragm

- Normal quiet breathing is accomplished almost entirely by the movement of diaphragm.
  - **Inspiration** – Contraction of **diaphragm.**
  - **Expiration** – Relaxation of **diaphragm** and elastic recoiling of the lungs, chest wall and abdominal muscles compress the lungs to expel the air.
- During heavy breathing, **abdominal muscles** contracts pushing the abdominal contents upwards compressing the lungs.

Change in anteroposterior diameter of the chest wall

- Muscles of inspiration and expiration causes movement of the chest wall.
- **Muscles of inspiration:**
  - **External intercostals*** are the important muscles of inspiration.
  - **Sternocleidomastoid*** muscles, **anterior serrate*** and **scalene*** are the other inspiratory muscles.
- **Muscles of expiration: Abdominal recti*** and **internal intercostals***.

Ans: (c) Abdominal muscles

Ref: *Guyton and Hall Textbook of Medical Physiology, 13th edition, Page 567*

9. Normal Carotid intima-media thickness (CIMT) is:

(a) 0.7 mm
(b) 2 mm
(c) 1.5 mm
(d) 1 mm

Explanation:

Carotid Intima-media thickness (CIMT)

- Measure of the combined thickness of intima and media layers of carotid artery. It is most commonly assessed by **B-mode ultrasound.**
- In healthy middle-aged adults, CIMT values between **0.6 and 0.7 mm** have been considered normal. CIMT of 1 mm or more has been associated with significant increased absolute risk of **CHD**.
- Increase in CIMT occurs due to **hypertrophy of intimal or medial layers** or both.
- Mechanisms that increase CIMT are also the factors responsible for development and progression of **atherosclerosis**.
- Assessment of CIMT is considered as method to detect **primordial atherosclerosis**.

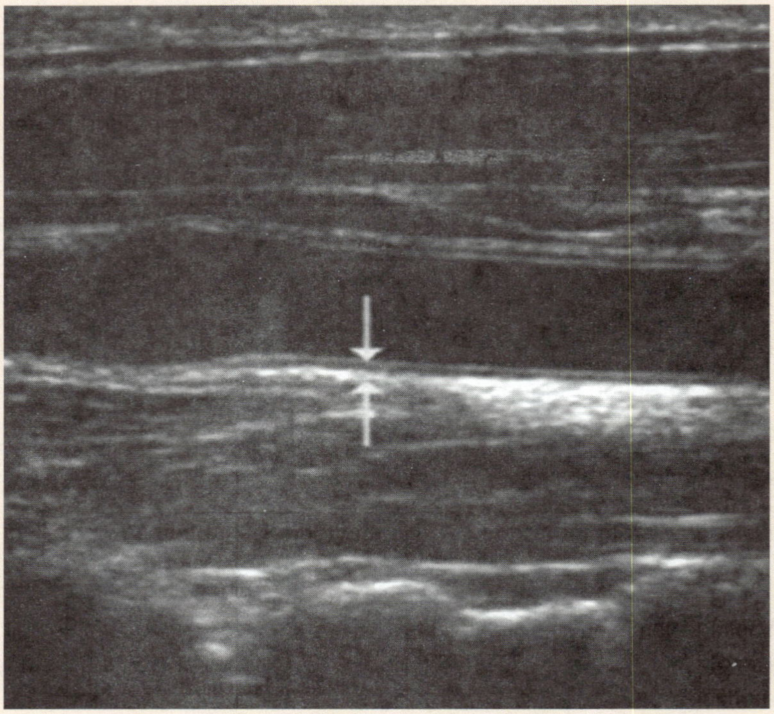

Figure: Carotid Intima-media thickness (CIMT)

Ans: (a) 0.7 mm

Ref: *Kasliwal RR, Bansal M, Desai D, Sharma M. Carotid intima-media thickness: Current evidence, practices and Indian experience. Indian Journal of Endocrinology and Metabolism 2014 Jan; 18(1):13*

10. Cut off value of BNP to diagnose heart failure is:

(a) > 900 pg/mL (b) > 600 pg/mL

(c) >100 pg/mL (d) > 40 pg/mL

Explanation:

Brain Natriuretic Peptide (BNP)

- Brain Natriuretic peptide also called **B type Natriuretic peptide (BNP)** and N Terminal Pro B Type **NT Pro BNP** are the most frequently measured natriuretic peptides are useful biomarkers for diagnosis of **Heart Failure (HF).**
- BNP and NT-proBNP are synthesized by the **cardiomyocytes** in response to **wall stress** during **ventricular stretch**.
- The half-life of **BNP** is **20 mins** and **NT Pro BNP** is **90 minutes.**
- Natriuretic peptides are elevated in:
  - **Ventricular systolic and diastolic dysfunctions***
  - **Valvular heart disease***
  - **Pulmonary hypertension***
  - Ischemic heart disease
  - Atrial arrhythmias.
- Elevated natriuretic peptides are also seen in **renal failure* and sepsis***.

- A cut off value of more than **100 pg/mL** concentration of BNP was highly accurate for diagnosis of **acute decompensated heart failure**. Similarly more than **900 pg/mL** was more accurate with **NT Pro BNP**.

Ans: (c) > 100 pg/ml

Ref: *Douglas Zipes et al., Braunwald's Heart Disease A Textbook of Cardiovascular Medicine, 11th edition*

11. Waves seen in EEG during stage 4–NREM period of sleep is:

(a) Alpha (b) Beta

(c) Delta (d) Theta

Explanation:

Non–REM Sleep (Slow Wave Sleep) – 4 stages

- **Stage 1**
  - Beta to alpha rhythm
- **Stage 2**
  - Amplitude increases
  - **Sleep spindle** (12-14 Hz; 50 **µ**V; for about 2 Seconds) and **K complexes** (high amplitude)
- **Stage 3**
  - High amplitude; low frequency
- **Stage 4**
  - Delta rhythm
- **Autonomic and visceral changes**
  - ↓ heart rate and BP
  - ↓ body temperature
  - Slow regular respiration
  - ↑ GI activity
  - ↓ muscle tone
  - No rapid eye movement

Ans: (c) Delta

Ref: *Reticular Formation, EEG and Sleep. In: Textbook of Medical Physiology, Ahuja Publishing House 2007;119:895*

12. Hormonal secretions are tightly controlled by the time of day sensed by an inbuilt biological clock in human body. This rhythmic secretion is controlled by:

(a) Supra optic nuclei (b) Posterolateral nucleus

(c) Ventro-lateral nucleus (d) Supra chiasmatic nucleus

Explanation:

- The inbuilt biological clock controlling secretion of hormones is known as **Circadian rhythm**. It is dependent on the **supra-chiasmatic nuclei (SCN)** located bilaterally above the **optic chiasm of brain.**

Function of Hypothalamus

Region	Area	Nucleus	Function
Anterior	Medial	Medial preoptic nucleus	• Regulates the release of **gonadotropic** hormones from the adenohypophysis • Contains the sexually dimorphic nucleus, which releases **GnRH**, differential development between sexes is based upon in utero testosterone levels
		Supraoptic nucleus (SO)	• **Vasopressin** release
		Paraventricular nucleus* (PV)	• **Thyrotropin-releasing** hormone release • **Corticotropin-releasing** hormone release • **Oxytocin** release
		Anterior hypothalamic nucleus (AH)	• **Thermoregulation** • Panting • **Sweating** • Thyrotropin inhibition
		Suprachiasmatic nucleus (SC)	• **Circadian rhythms**
	Lateral	Lateral preoptic nucleus	
		Lateral nucleus (LT)	• **Thirst** and **hunger**
		Part of supraoptic nucleus (SO)	
Tuberal	Medial	**Dorsomedial hypothalamic nucleus (DM)**	• **Blood Pressure** • **Heart Rate** • **GI stimulation**
		Ventromedial nucleus (VM)	• **Satiety** • **Neuroendocrine** control
		Arcuate nucleus (AR)	• **Growth hormone-releasing hormone (GHRH)** • **Feeding** • **Dopamine**
	Lateral	**Lateral nucleus (LT)**	• **Thirst** and hunger
		Lateral tuberal nuclei	
Posterior	Medial	**Mammillary nuclei** (part of mammillary bodies) (MB)	• **Memory**
		Posterior nucleus (PN)	• Increase blood pressure • **Pupillary** dilation • **Shivering** • Vasopressin release
	Lateral	Lateral nucleus (LT)	

Ans: (d) Supra chiasmatic nucleus

Ref: *W F Ganong, Central and Peripheral Neurophysiology. In: Review of Medical Physiology, 24th edition, California: McGraw-Hill Companies; 2012, Page 278*

13. In a measurement of cardiac output using the Fick principle, the O_2 concentrations of mixed venous and arterial blood are 16 and 20 ml· 100 ml-1, respectively, and the O_2 consumption is 300 ml·min-1. The cardiac output in liters·min-1 is:

(a) 5 (b) 8
(c) 9 (d) 7.5

Explanation:

- Cardiac output is the amount of blood ejected by each ventricle per minute. Normal cardiac output is 5-6 Lit/minute.
- Cardiac index is cardiac output/body surface area.
- Factors such as exercise, anxiety, emotion, excitement, pregnancy, etc., increase cardiac output.
- **Methods of measurement of cardiac output:** Fick's principle, indicator dilution method, Thermodilution method, ballistocardiography, Echocardiography, etc.

Fick's Principle:

- The Fick principle states that the cardiac output is equal to the oxygen consumption divided by the arterial-venous oxygen concentration difference.

$$\textit{Cardiac output} = \frac{\textit{Oygen absorbed per minute by the lungs (ml per min)}}{\textit{Arteriovenous } O_2 \textit{ difference (mL per Lit of blood)}}$$

- Here,
  - Oxygen consumption is 300 ml per minute.
  - Arterioveous difference is (20 - 16) ml·100 ml-1 or (200 – 160) ml·liter-1.
  - Therefore, the cardiac output is equal to 300/(200 – 160) or 7.5 liters·min-1.

Ans: (d) 7.5

Ref: *Ganong, 25th edition, Page 543*

14. Formula to calculate minute ventilation volume:

(a) TV × RR (b) FiO_2/PEEP
(c) TV × (RR–dead space) (d) TV + (RR–dead space)

Explanation:

MINUTE VENTILATION AND ALVEOLAR VENTILATION

- **Minute ventilation or Respiratory Minute Volume** is the amount of **air inspired or expired per minute**. It is calculated as **tidal volume times breaths per minute,** i.e.,
  - **Minute Ventilation = Tidal Volume × Respiratory Rate**
  - Normal Minute Ventilation volume is about **6 L** (MV = 500 mL × 12 breaths per minute)
- **Alveolar Ventilation** is the **amount of fresh gas reaching the alveoli**. It takes part in gas exchange.
  - **Alveolar Ventilation = (Tidal Volume – Dead Space) × Respiratory Rate**
  - Normal Alveolar Ventilation is about **4.2 L** [Alveolar Ventilation = (500-150) × 12]

Dead Space

- The anatomic dead space is the volume of air present in the conducting zone that does not take part in gaseous exchange. It can be measured by **Single breath Nitrogen Technique.**

- The physiologic dead space includes both anatomical dead space and alveolar dead space. It is calculated by **Bohr's equation.**
- In healthy individuals anatomical dead space and physiological dead space are equal.
- Physiological dead space is higher in conditions such as Emphysema, Bronchiectasis, etc.

Ans: (a) TV × RR

Ref: *John B West, Respiratory Physiology: The Essentials, 9th edition, Page 20*

BIOCHEMISTRY

1. Rapoport Luebering cycle shift O_2 dissociation curve to right because of:

(a) 2,3 DPG
(b) 1,3 BPG
(c) 3 phosphoglycerate
(d) 1,6 fructose bisphosphate

Explanation:

Rapoport Luebering Cycle

- Takes place in RBCs.
- Bisphosphoglycerate mutase converts 1,3 Bis phosphoglycerate to 2,3 Bisphosphoglycerate (2,3 BPG).
- Removal of phosphate by phosphatase to form 3-Phosphoglycerate.

Significance of 2,3 BPG

- Combines with Hb, reduces the affinity towards oxygen...... increased supply of oxygen to tissues.
- Increased supply of oxygen to tissues in hypoxic conditions as conc of 2,3 BPG increases.
- No ATP generated, hence shunt pathway of glycolysis to waste the energy not required.

Oxygen Dissociation Curve

- A plot of % saturation of Hb with O_2 measured at different partial pressures of oxygen (pO_2).
- O_2 saturation curve for Hb is Sigmoid.
- The steep slope of the ODC over the range of oxygen concentrations that occur between the lungs and the tissues permits Hb to carry and deliver oxygen efficiently from sites of high to sites of low pO_2.

There are four primary regulators, each of which has a negative impact:

- CO_2
- Hydrogen ion (H^+)
- Chloride ion (Cl^-)
- 2,3-bisphosphoglycerate (2,3-BPG)

The curve shifts to the **RIGHT** (representing a **decrease in affinity** for O_2) in:

- Acute acidosis
- Increase in pCO_2
- Increase in temperature
- Increase in 2,3-bisphosphoglycerate

The curve shifts to the **LEFT** (representing an **increase in affinity** for O_2):

- Acute alkalosis
- Decrease in $p(CO_2)$
- Decrease in temperature
- Decrease in 2,3-bisphosphoglycerate

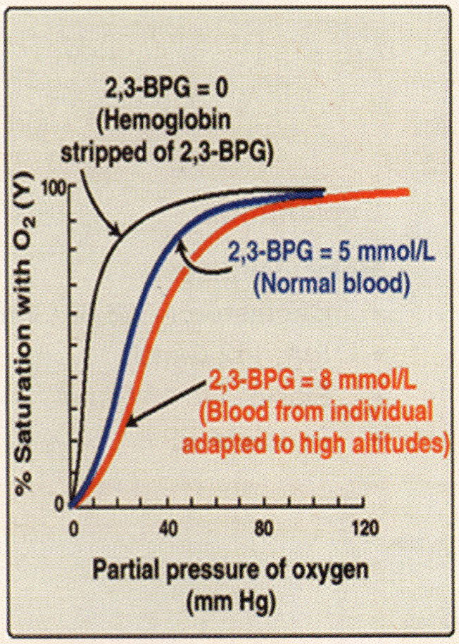

Figure: Effect of 2,3 BPG on oxygen dissociation curve

Ans: (a) 2, 3 DPG

Ref: *Lippincott's Illustrated Reviews, Biochemistry, 5th edition, Chapter-8, Page 101 and Chapter-3, Page 32*

2. Ketone bodies may be seen in:

(a) Diabetes mellitus
(b) Pancreatitis
(c) Obesity
(d) Myocardial infarction

Explanation:

- **Diabetes mellitus is a metabolic syndrome characterised by hyperglycemia due to absolute or relative deficiency of insulin.**

Decreased glucose transport due to insulin insufficiency

↓

Increased Lipolysis

↓

Increased free fatty acids

↓

Increased beta oxidation

↓

Ketogenesis

↓

Ketonemia/ketonuria

Ans: (a) Diabetes mellitus

Ref: *Lippincott's Illustrated Reviews, Biochemistry, 5th edition, Chapter-25, Page 334*

3. Arrange according to molecular size:

(a) Platelets>cholesterol>fibrin>IgA
(b) Cholesterol >Platelets>IgA>fibrin
(c) Cholesterol>IgA>Fibrin>Platelets
(d) IgA>cholesterol>platelets>fibrin

Explanation:

Molecular Sizes:

- **Cholesterol**–386.65 G/mol
- **IgA**–162 G/mol
- **Fibrin**–145.16 G/mol
- **Platelets**–$29 \times 1.66 \times 10^{-24.}$ mg

Ans: (c) Cholesterol>IgA>Fibrin>Platelets

Ref: *Multiple Sources*

4. Vitamins playing an important role in citric acid cycle:

(a) Thiamine, riboflavin, niacin, lipoic acid
(b) Thiamine, biotin, riboflavin, pantothenic acid
(c) Thiamine, pyridoxine, riboflavin, niacin, pantothenic
(d) Thiamine mecobalamin, pantothenic acid

Explanation:

Coenzymes of various vitamins involved in TCA cycle as follows:

- **Thiamine**: thiamine pyrophosphate (TPP)
- **Riboflavin**: Flavin adenine dinucleotide (FAD)
- **Niacin**: Niacin adenine dinucleotide (NAD)
- Lipoic acid

Pyruvate is converted to **Acetyl CoA** by **pyruvate dehydrogenase**, which is a multi enzyme complex. The vitamins associated with these enzymes is given in the table below:

Enzyme	Abbreviated	Prosthetic Group
Pyruvate Dehydrogenase	E_1	Thiamine pyrophosphate (TPP)
Dihydrolipoyl Transacetylase	E_2	Lipoamide
Dihydrolipoyl Dehydrogenase	E_1	FAD

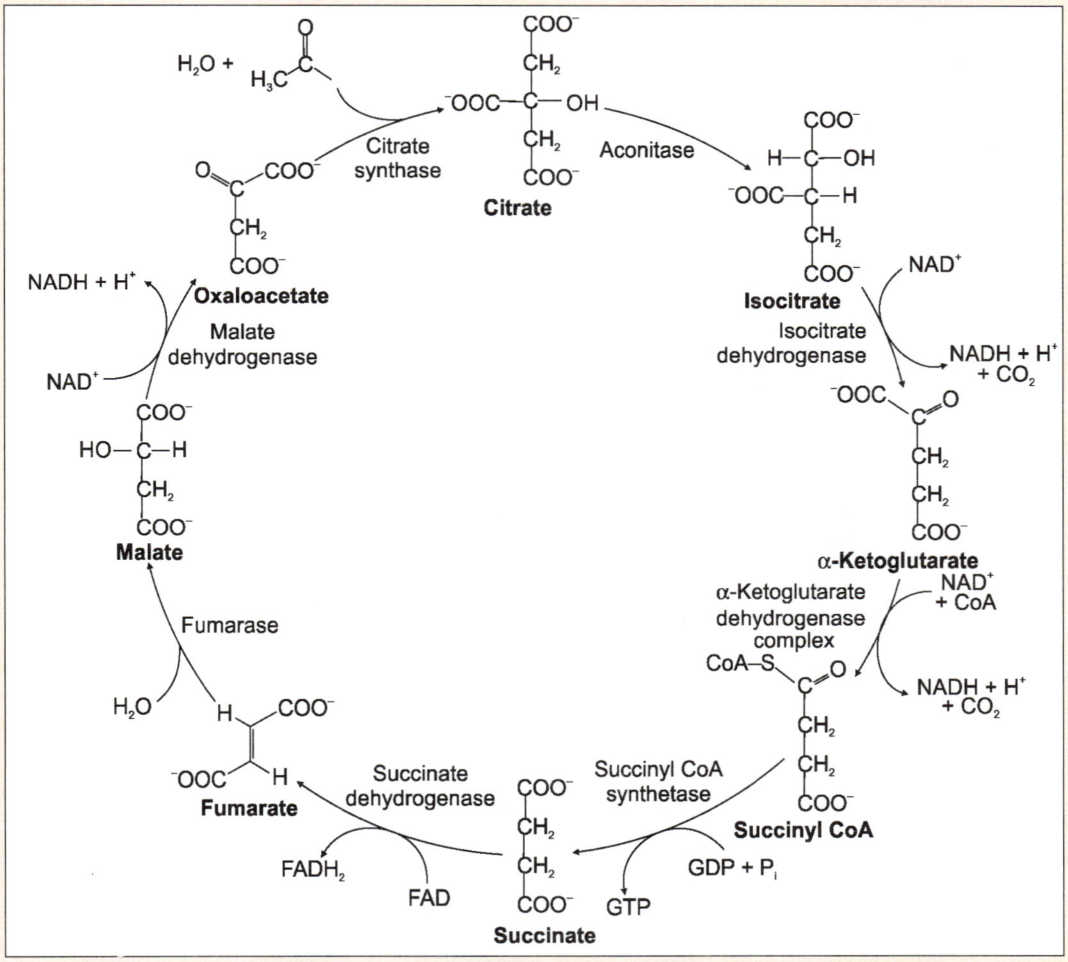

Figure: TCA cycle

Ans: (a) Thiamine, riboflavin, niacin, lipoic acid

Ref: *Lippincott's Illustrated Reviews, Biochemistry, 5th edition, Chapter-9, Page 109-113*

5. Dimercaprol inhibits:

(a) ETC complex 1
(b) ETC complex 2
(c) ETC complex 3
(d) ETC complex 4

Explanation:

COMPONENTS OF ELECTRON TRANSPORT CHAIN (ETC)

- **Complex - I**
  - **NADH dehydrogenase** complex or **NADH – CoQ Reductase.**
  - It is a Flavoprotein containing **FMN Fe-S** Protein.
- **Complex - II**
  - Electrons from FADH enters into ETC through CoQ.
  - **Succinate dehydrogenase.**
  - FADH2 are transferring electrons to this complex.
- **Complex - III**
  - Complex III is also known as **Cytochrome Reductase**.
  - It is **cytochrome b and c1.**
  - It is composed of Fe-S-Protein + Heme as prosthetic group.
- **Complex - IV**
  - It is also known as **cytochrome oxidase.**
  - It is containing **cytochrome a + a3.**
  - Besides iron in cytochrome, it contains two copper ions.
- **Complex - V (ATP synthase)**
  - ATP synthase or complex V.
  - It is also known as **F1 – Fo ATPase.**
  - It looks like a **'lollipop'.**
  - It has two functional subunits – **F1 and Fo**.
  - 'o' styands for oligomycin.

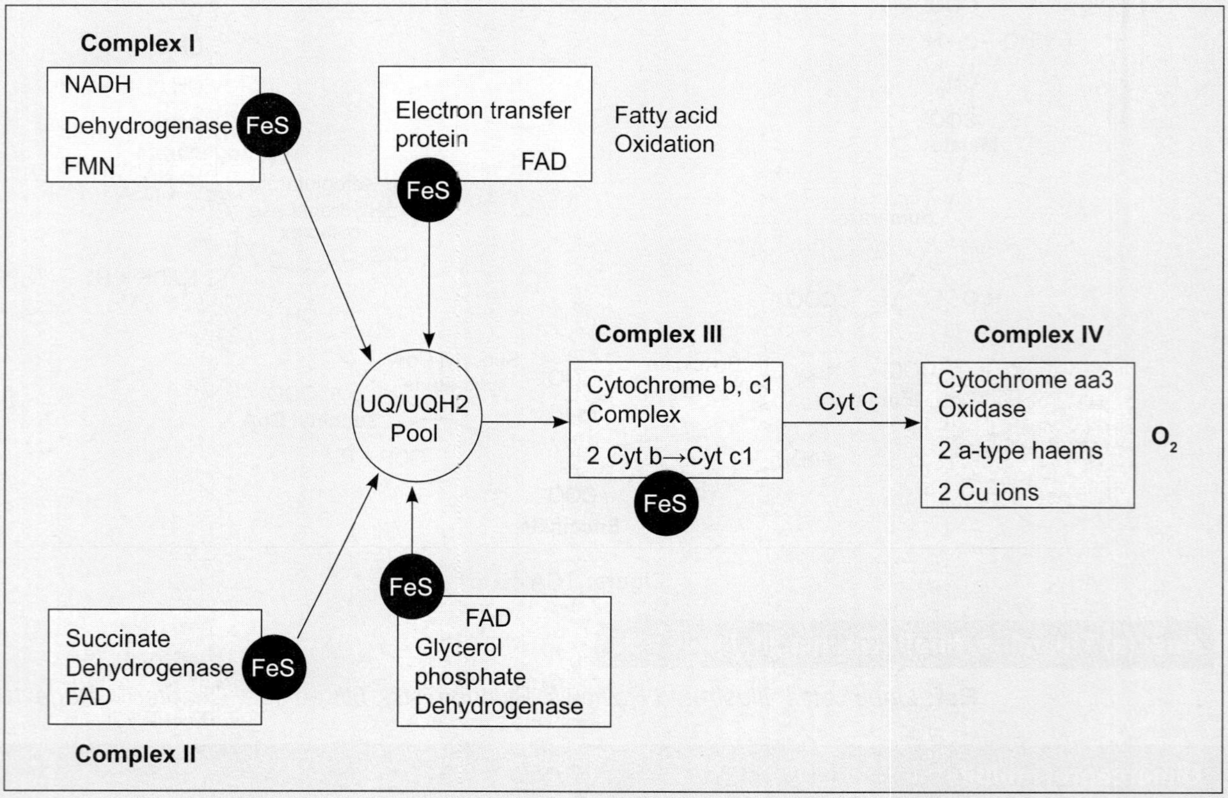

Figure: Electron transport chain

Inhibitors of ETC

Site	Complex	Inhibitor
Site-I	***Complex I***	Barbiturate Piericidin A Rotenone
Site-II	***Complex III***	Antimycin A BAL Dimercaprol
Site III	***Complex IV***	Azide Carbon monoxide Cyanide Hydrogen sulphide

Ans: (c) ETC complex 3

Ref: *Lippincott's Illustrated Reviews, Biochemistry, 5th edition, Chapter-6, Page 75-76*

6. Enzyme deficient in Hyperammonemia type 1:

(a) Ornithine transcarbamoylase
(b) Arginase
(c) Carbamoyl phosphate synthase I
(d) Arginosuccinate synthase

Explanation:

Urea Cycle Disorders:

Disorder	Inheritance	Enzyme defect	Clinical Manifestations
Hyperammonemia I	Inborn defect	**CPS I**	• Ammonia toxicity • Ataxia • Protein intolerance
Hyperammonemia II	X-linked deficiency	**OTC**	• Ammonia toxicity • Increases levels of glutamine, ornithine and ammonia in the blood
Citrullinemia	Double recessive	**Argininosuccinate synthase**	• Increased levels of citrulline in the blood • Hyperammonemia • Mental retardation
Argininosuccinic aciduria	Double recessive	**Argininosuccinate lyase**	• High levels of argininosuccinate in blood, urine and CSF • Mental retardation • Friable tufted hair
Arginemia		**Arginase**	• Increased Arg levels in the blood, CSF and brain • Increased levels of amino acids transported by the COAL transporter

Ans: (c) Carbamoyl phosphate synthase I

Ref: *Harper's Illustrated Biochemistry, 28th edition*

7. During vigorous exercise, which of the following is released from the muscles?

(a) Alanine
(b) Glutamine
(c) Branched keto acid
(d) Asparagine

Explanation:

Glucose-alanine cycle happens during **fasting.** It is exemplified in **vigorous exercise.**

As illustrated in the figure:

- During **fasting or strenuous exercise**, **muscle breaks down proteins** to **amino acids**.
- The nitrogen from the amino acids is **transaminated** to **pyruvate** to produce **alanine**. This **alanine** is released into the blood stream.
- **Liver** takes up the alanine and converts back to **pyruvate** by **transamination**.
- **Pyruvate** is **glucogenic**.

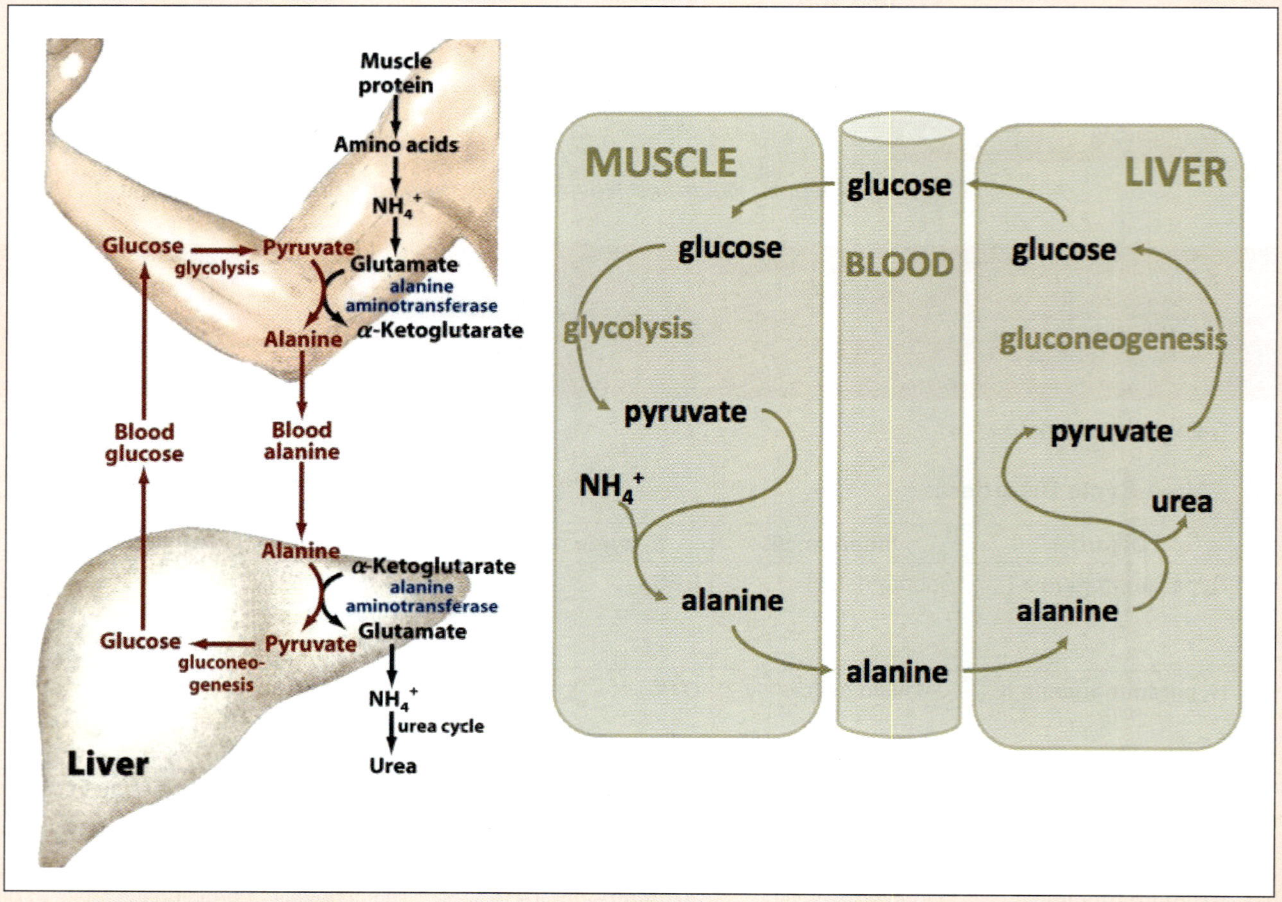

Biochemical changes seen in vigorous exercise:

- ↑ CK-MB, AST, ALT in plasma
- ↓ Na^+, K^+, Glucose plasma
- Proteinuria

Other options:

- **Glutamine** helps in **ammonia detoxification** from **brain**.
- **Branched keto acids** are excretec in **Maple syrup urine disease**.
- **Asparagine** is a **non-essential amino acid** that can be **synthesised** from **aspartate**.

Ans: (a) Alanine

Ref: *Harper, 30th edition, Page191, Fig.19-5*

8. Ketone bodies not utilised by:

(a) Brain
(b) RBC
(c) Heart
(d) Skeletal muscle

Explanation:

*"Unlike **fatty acids**, **ketone bodies** can be used by the **brain** (but **not** by cells, such as **red blood cells**, that **lack mitochondria**) and thus are important **fuels** during a **fast**. The liver lacks the ability to degrade ketone bodies, and so synthesizes them specifically for the peripheral tissues."*

Ref: Lippincott's Biochemistry*, 3rd edition, Page 486*

Substrate utilized by various organs in different states

Organ	Fed State	Fasting	Starvation
Brain	Glucose	Glucose	Ketone bodies
Heart	Fatty acid	Fatty acid	Ketone bodies
Liver	Glucose	Fatty acid	Amino acid
Muscles	Glucose	Fatty acid	Fatty acid

KETOLYSIS

- Utilization of ketone bodies
- **Site**:
  - **Mitochondria**
  - **Extra hepatic tissue**
- **Tissues**
  - **Heart**
  - **Brain (especially when starving)**
  - **Skeletal muscle**
  - **Renal cortex**
- **Ketones** are **NOT** utilized by:
  - **RBC** – Since it does **NOT** contain **Mitochondria**
  - **Liver** – Since it does **NOT** contain **thiophorase enzyme.**

Note:

- **Liver** is the **ONLY organ** which produces **ketone bodies** and releases into **blood**, but it **lacks the enzyme** responsible (**Thiophorase**) for their degradation and utilization. This is the reason why liver does not utilize ketone bodies.

Ans: (b) RBC

Ref: *Harper's Illustrated Biochemistry, 27th edition, Page 190 and Lippincott's Biochemistry, 3rd edition, Page 486*

PHARMACOLOGY

1. Bile acid resins causes.....% decrease in LDL and ....% increase in HDL.

(a) 10-15% and 3-5%
(b) 15-25% and 3-5%
(c) 3-5% and 15-30%
(d) 25-35% and 5-10%

Explanation:

Bile Acid Sequestrants/Resins

- Includes **Cholestyramine, Colestipol and Colesevelam**
- Effect of **Bile acid resins** on plasma lipids:
  - ↓ LDL by 15-25%
  - ↑ HDL by 3-5%
  - Effect on TG levels is negligible
- Effect of **Statins** on **plasma lipids:**
  - ↓ LDL by 20-55%
  - ↑ HDL by 5-15%
  - ↓ TG by 10-35%
- Effect of **fibrates** on **plasma lipids:**
  - ↓ LDL by 5-15%
  - ↑ HDL by 10-20%
  - ↓ TG by 20-50%
- Effect of **nicotinic acid** on **plasma lipids:**
  - ↓ LDL by 15-25%
  - ↑ HDL by 20-35%
  - ↓ TG by 20-50%

Ans: (b) 15-25% and 3-5%

Ref: *Tripathi KD, Essentials of Medical Pharmacology, 8th edition, New Delhi, Jaypee Brothers Medical Publishers, 2019, Page 685*

2. Which of the following statements is false regarding bedaquiline?

(a) Inhibits mycobacterial cell wall synthesis
(b) Causes QT prolongation
(c) Half life is very long
(d) Indicated for MDR TB

Explanation:

BEDAQUILINE

- MOA: Inhibits **mycobacterial ATP synthase***
- **Mechanism of Resistance:**
  - **Mutation** in the **ATP synthase enzyme**
  - **Drug efflux**

- **Pharmacokinetics:**
  - Good oral absorption
  - Plasma protein binding: **High**
  - Metabolism: **Liver [CY3A4]**
  - Terminal $t_{1/2}$: **Long [160 days]**
  - Excretion: **Feces**
- **Indications:**
  - Pulmonary MDR-TB in adults
- Always should be combined with at least three/four other susceptible antitubercular drugs as per culture sensitivity pattern to enhance the efficacy and reduce the resistance pattern.
- **Dosage and Regimen:**
  - Initially 400 mg/day for 2 weeks
  - Then 200 mg three times/week for next 22 weeks
  - Total duration of therapy is 24 weeks
- **Adverse effects:**
  - Mild: Nausea, headache, arthralgia
  - ECG changes: QTc prolongation
  - Hepatotoxicity

Ans: (a) Inhibits mycobacterial cell wall synthesis

Ref: *Tripathi KD, Essentials of Medical Pharmacology, 8th edition, New Delhi, Jaypee Brothers Medical Publishers, 2019, Page 822*

3. Raxibacumab is used in:

(a) Anthrax (b) Pontiac fever

(c) Listeria (d) Clostridium

Explanation:

RAXIBACUMAB

- Human monoclonal antibody against ***Bacillus anthracis***
- Monoclonal antibody targeting the **protective antigen (PA) component** of the **lethal toxin** of **Bacillus anthracis** and is being developed for the **treatment of inhalational anthrax**
- Approved for use in both Adult and pediatric patients
  - In combination with appropriate antibacterial drugs
  - Prophylaxis of inhalational anthrax when alternative therapies are not available
  - Treatment of **inhalational anthrax** with Raxibacumab injection (FDA approved)
- Adults Dose: 40 mg/kg raxibacumab
- Adverse effects
  - Headaches
  - URI
  - Nausea
  - Pain in limbs
  - Pruritis

Ans: (a) Anthrax

Ref: *https://www.accessdata.fda.gov/drugsatfda_docs/label/2012/125349s000lbl.pdf*

4. Which of the following statement is true regarding Atazanavir?

(a) Effective against only HIV-1

(b) Resistance is due to mutation in codon 50 isoleucine to valine substitution

(c) ↓ Cholesterol and TG levels

(d) Combination with ritonavir do not have any advantage

Explanation:

ATAZANAVIR

- **Protease inhibitor** active against both **HIV-1 and HIV-2***
- Mechanism of resistance is due to:
  - Mutation in HIV protease **codon 50,** with isoleucine to **leucine substitution**
- Pharmacokinetics:
  - **Good oral absorption** with peak serum concentration in **2 hours**
  - Absorption is food and pH dependent
  - Absorption is **increased** with **food**
  - ↓ in pH can ↓ the absorption of atazanavir
  - Metabolism: **Liver [CYP3A4]**
  - $t_{1/2}$: **7 Hours**
  - Plasma protein binding: 86%
  - CSF concentration: Less than 3% of plasma concentration
  - Seminal fluid concentration: Excellent
- **Adverse effects:**
  - **Unconjugated hyperbilirubinemia**
  - **Cholecystitis, cholelithiasis**, cholestasis and other hepatic function abnormalities
  - GIT: Nausea, diarrhea
  - Carbohydrate intolerance/(↓) insulin sensitivity
  - **Drug interactions:**
    - Atazanavir substrate as well as moderate inhibitor of CYP3A4
    - Levels of atazanavir are affected by potent inducers (Ex. Rifampin)
    - Atazanavir can alter the plasma levels of other CYP3A4 substrates
    - Ritonavir (↑) the concentration of atazanavir and this interaction is beneficial in therapeutic dosing and efficacy
- (↓) Fasting TG and cholesterol levels
- **Clinical Indications:**
  - HIV-1 and HIV-2 infections
  - Also approved in children **less than 6 years of age**

Ans: (c) ↓ Cholesterol and TG levels

Ref: *Flexner C, Antiretroviral Agents and Treatment of HIV Infection, In: Brunton L, Chabner B, Knollman B Editors, Goodman and Gillman's The Pharmacological Basis of Therapeutics, 12th edition, New York: McGraw-Hill; 2011, Page 1652-1653*

5. Mechanism of resistance of tetracyclines is due to:

(a) Drug efflux mechanism
(b) Both drug influx and drug efflux mechanisms
(c) DNA methylation
(d) Cell wall alteration

Explanation:

Tetracyclines:

- Broad spectrum antimicrobial agents
- **Mechanism of resistance** of tetracyclines is due to:
  - (↓) Drug influx into target cells
  - (↑) Drug efflux
  - Mutation in ribosomal proteins
  - Enzymatic inactivation

Tigecycline:

- **Glycylcyclines** with improved efficacy against tetracyclines resistant microorganisms; this improved efficacy is due to:
  - **Glycylamido** moiety in **tigecycline** (↓) affinity towards **drug efflux proteins** and thus do not susceptible to resistance by this mechanism.
  - Improved and better binding of tigecycline with ribosomal proteins also enhances its efficacy without much susceptible to resistance mediated through mutation of ribosomal proteins.

Ans: (b) Both drug influx and drug efflux mechanisms

Ref: *MacDougall C, Chambers HF, Protein Synthesis Inhibitors and Miscellaneous Antibacterial Agents. In: Brunton L, Chabner B, Knollman B Editors. Goodman and Gillman's The Pharmacological Basis of Therapeutics, 12th edition, New York: McGraw-Hill, 2011, Page 1652-1653*

6. Initial drug to start with newly detected Hypertension in an 42 years old male with calcium stones (nephrolithiasis) is:

(a) Furosemide
(b) Spironolactone
(c) Atenolol
(d) Thiazides

Explanation:

- **Thiazides:**
  - Thiazides **enhances Ca^{2+} reabsorption**
  - Hence very useful in treatment of recurrent calcium kidney stones caused due to hypercalciuria
- **Furosemide:**
  - Loop diuretic
  - Loop diuretics **enhances Ca^{2+} excretion** through **kidney**
  - **Hypercalciuria** caused due to **loop diuretics** may enhance the formation of **calcium kidney stones**

Ans: (d) Thiazides

Ref: *Tripathi KD, Essentials of Medical Pharmacology, 8th edition, New Delhi: Jaypee Brothers Medical Publishers, 2019, Page 631*

7. Diplopia with dizziness are side effects of which of the following drug combination?

(a) Phenytoin and carbamazepine
(b) Lamotrigene and carbamazepine
(c) Gabapentin with phenytoin
(d) Valproate and topiramate

Explanation:

ADRS OF PHENYTOIN

- **At therapeutic plasma concentration**
  - **Gum hypertrophy***
  - Facial: **Acne, hirsutism**
  - Hypersensitivity reactions
  - **Osteomalacia*** and **megaloblastic anemia***
- **Above therapeutic plasma concentration**
  - **Cerebellar symptoms*:** Vertigo, diplopia, ataxia
  - Drowsiness, mental clouding
  - GIT: Nausea, vomiting, epigastric pain

ADRS OF CARBAMAZEPINE

- **Neurotoxicity*:** Dizziness, diplopia, vertigo, ataxia
- GIT, Nausea, vomiting, diarrhea
- Hypersensitivity reactions
- **Dilutional hyponatraemia***

Ans: (a) Phenytoin and carbamazepine

Ref: *Tripathi KD, Essentials of Medical Pharmacology, 8th edition, New Delhi, Jaypee Brothers Medical Publishers, 2019, Page 441*

8. Dose of fosfomycin in a 40 years patient who is weighing 60 kg:

(a) 6 gm single dose
(b) 6 mg/kg single dose
(c) 3 gm single dose
(d) 3 mg/kg single dose

Explanation:

Fosfomycin

- Antimicrobial agent acts by **inhibiting cell wall synthesis***
- **Pharmacokinetics**:
  - Absorption: Good
  - Bioavailability = 30-60%
  - Distribution: avd = 2 L/kg; Attains higher concentration in urine and CSF
  - PPB = Less than 3%
- **Clinical indications:**
  - UTI
  - **Prostatitis**

- **Dose:**
  - 3 g single dose PO for UTI
  - 3 g PO every 3 days for 21 days for prostatitis
- **Adverse effects:**
  - GIT: Nausea, vomiting, epigastric discomfort, diarrhea
  - Headache, dizziness
  - Rashes, pruritus

Ans: (c) 3 gm single dose

Ref: *BMJ Open 2013;3: e004157*

9. Which statin is not metabolized by CYP3A4?

(a) Lovastatin (b) Simvastatin
(c) Atorvastatin (d) Pravastatin

Explanation:

STATINS

- **HMG-CoA reductase inhibitors** used for **hypercholesterolemia and dyslipidemias**
- Statins include **atorvastatin, lovastatin, simvastatin, pravastatin, fluvastatin, rosuvastatin** etc
- Statins primarily metabolized by **CYP3A4/A5:**
  - Atorvastatin, lovastatin, simvastatin
- **Fluvastatin metabolism:**
  - CYP2C9 (50 - 80%)
  - CYP3A4 and CYP2C8 (20 - 50%)
- **Pravastatin metabolism:**
  - **NOT** metabolized by **CYP system** and is excreted **unchanged in the urine***
- Other statins which are **NOT** extensively metabolized by **CYP3A4** include:
  - Fluvastatin and rosuvastatin

Ans: (d) Pravastatin

Ref: *Bersot TP, Drug Therapy for Hypercholesterolemia and Dyslipidemia, In: Brunton L, Chabner B, Knollman B, Editors. Goodman and Gillman's The Pharmacological Basis of Therapeutics, 12th edition, New York: McGraw-Hill, 2011, Page 897*

10. Acetylcholine receptors has 5 subunits:

(a) α_2, β_1, δ and κ (b) α_1, β_2, δ and κ
(c) α_2, β_1, δ and ε (d) α_1, β_2, δ and ε

Explanation:

Acetylcholine

- It is a **neurotransmitter** at **preganglionic sympathetic** as well as **parasympathetic fibers** and at **postganglionic parasympathetic fibers.**

- Ach acts on two types of receptors:
  - Muscarinic
  - Nicotinic
- Major Ach muscarinic receptors include **M_1, M_2, M_3, M_4** and **M_5**
- Major Ach nicotinic receptors include **N_m** and **N_n**
- ACh muscarinic receptors are **GPCRs,** where nicotinic are ligand gated ion channels
- The structure of Ach nicotinic receptors is a **pentamer:**
  - N_m: $(\alpha_1)_2\beta_1\varepsilon\delta$ (Adults) and $(\alpha_1)_2\beta_1\gamma\delta$ (Fetal)
  - N_n: $(\alpha_3)_2(\beta_4)_3$
  - CNS: $(\alpha_4)_2(\beta_4)_3$ and $(\alpha_7)_5$

Ans: (c) α_2, β_1, δ and ε

Ref: *Westfall TC, Westfall DP, Neurotransmission: The Autonomic and Somatic Motor Nervous Systems. In: Brunton L, Chabner B, Knollman B editors. Goodman and Gillman's The Pharmacological Basis of Therapeutics, 12th edition, New York: McGraw-Hill, 2011, Page 191*

11. Which drug has anti-inflammatory and also has immune-modulator actions?

(a) Fluoroquinolones (b) Macrolides

(c) Tetracyclines (d) Acyclovir

Explanation:

- **Azithromycin (A), roxithromycin (R), erythromycin (E), and clarithromycin (C)** are commonly used in dermatology practice for their immunomodulatory and anti-inflammatory potential.

OTHER IMMUNOMODULATOR DRUGS

A. Immunosuppressants

- **Glucocorticoids**
- **Calcineurin inhibitors** – Tacrolimus
- **Proliferation signal inhibitors** – Sirolimus (rapamycin), Everolimus
- **Purine synthesis inhibitor** – Mycophenolate mofetil
- **Antimetabolites** – Azathioprine
- **Other Cytotoxic agents** – Cyclophosphamide, chlorambucil and methotrexate
- **Leflunomide**
- **Thalidomide**
- **Monoclonal Antibodies***
- **Co-stimulation inhibitors** – Abatacept (Rheumatoid arthritis) and belatacept (Preventing rejection in Renal transplant recipients)
- **IL-1 inhibitors** – Anakinra
- **Others** – Nintedanib (Idiopathic pulmonary fibrosis), Apremilast (Psoriasis)

B. Immunostimulators

- **Levamisole**
- **BCG**
- **Cytokines** – Aldesleukin (IL-2 analogue), Filgrastim (recombinant G-CSF) and sargramostim (recombinant GM-CSF)

- **Thalidomide**
- **Imiquimod**

Ans: (b) Macrolides

Ref: *Indian J Dermatol 2016;61:469-81*

12. The least common side effect of fluoroquinolones is:

(a) Abdominal discomfort
(b) Hypoglycemia
(c) QT prolongation
(d) Hallucinations

Explanation:

FLUOROQUINOLONES

- Antimicrobial agents acts by **inhibiting DNA gyrase***
- Adverse effects:
  - **Common** (3 -17%):
    - **GIT related** (nausea, vomiting, and/or abdominal discomfort)
    - **CNS related** (0.9 -11%): Mild headache and dizziness
  - Individual drug related:
    - **C. difficile colitis** (Ciprofloxacin)
    - **Hypo- and hyperglycemia** (Gatifloxacin)
    - Theophylline toxicity (Ciprofloxacin and pefloxacin)
    - **QTc interval prolongation** (Sparfloxacin, gatifloxacin and moxifloxacin)
  - Others:
    - Rashes including photosensitivity
    - **Achilles tendon rupture or tendinitis***
  - Rare:
    - **Hallucinations,** delirium and seizures
    - Leukopenia, eosinophilia, and mild elevations in serum transaminases

Ans: (d) Hallucinations

Ref: *Petri WA, Sulfonamides, Trimethoprim–Sulfamethoxazole, Quinolones and Agents for Urinary Tract Infections. In: Brunton L, Chabner B, Knollman B editors. Goodman and Gillman's The Pharmacological Basis of Therapeutics, 12th edition, New York: McGraw-Hill, 2011, Page 1473 -1474*

13. Which of the following combinations can result in severe toxicity due to inhibition of Cytochrome 450 enzyme?

(a) Amiodarone + Cimetidine
(b) Carbamazepine + Phenytoin
(c) Atorvastatin + Itraconazole
(d) Phenytoin + Rifampin

Explanation:

Cytochrome P450 Enzymes

- These are essential for the metabolism of many medications.

- Although this class has more than 50 enzymes, six of them metabolize 90 percent of drugs, with the two most significant enzymes being CYP3A4 and CYP2D6.

Enzyme	Potent inhibitors	Potent inducers	Substrates
CYP1A2	• Amiodarone • Cimetidine • Ciprofloxacin • Fluvoxamine	• Carbamazepine • Phenobarbital • Rifampin • Tobacco	• Caffeine • Clozapine • Theophylline
CYP2C9	• Amiodarone • Fluconazole • Fluoxetine • Metronidazole • Ritonavir • Trimethoprim/ sulfamethoxazol	• Carbamazepine • Phenobarbital • Phenytoin • Rifampin	• Carvedilol • Celecoxib • Glipizide • Ibuprofen • Irbesartan • Losartan
CYP2C19	• Fluvoxamine • Isoniazid (INH) • Ritonavir	• Carbamazepine • Phenytoin • Rifampin	• Omeprazole • Phenobarbital • Phenytoin
CYP2D6	• Amiodarone • Cimetidine • Diphenhydramine • Fluoxetine • Paroxetine • Quinidine • Ritonavir • Terbinafine	• No significant inducers	• Amitriptyline • Carvedilol • Donepezil • Haloperidol • Metoprolol • Paroxetine • Risperidone • Tramadol
CYP3A4 and CYP3A5	• Clarithromycin • Diltiazem • Erythromycin • Grapefruit juice • Itraconazole • Ketoconazole • Nefazodone • Ritonavir • Telithromycin • Verapamil	• Carbamazepine • *Hypericum perforatum* (St. John's wort) • Phenobarbital • Phenytoin • Rifampin	• Alprazolam • Amlodipine • Atorvastatin • Cyclosporine • Diazepam • Estradiol • Simvastatin • Sildenafil • Verapamil • Zolpidem

Ans: (c) Atorvastatin + Itraconazole

Ref: *Am Fam Physician, 2007 Aug 1;76(3): 391-396*

14. Which of the following decreases defibrillation threshold?

(a) Amiodarone (b) Verapamil

(c) Sotalol (d) Diltiazem

Explanation:

- **Defibrillation threshold** indicates the minimum amount of energy needed to return normal rhythm to a heart that is beating in a cardiac dysrhythmia.

- Defibrillation threshold is a concept also applicable to **internal or implantable cardiac defibrillators**

Table: Effects of Antiarrhythmic Medications on Difibrillation Threshold

Increase	No change	Decrease
Amiodarone (chronic)	Beta blocker	Amiodarone (acute)
Atropine	Disopyramide	Sotalol
Diltiazem	Procainamide	Nifekalant
Verapamil	Propafenone	
Flecainide		

Ans: (c) Sotalol

Ref: *Arrhythmia and Electrophysiology Review 2018;7(4):288-93*

15. All are true regarding Isavuconazonium sulfate except:

(a) Effective against yeasts, molds and dimorphic fungi
(b) Acts through blocking cytoplasmic proteins
(c) Approved for aspergillosis and mucormycosis
(d) Devoid of nephrotoxicity

Explanation:

ISAVUCONAZONIUM SULFATE

- **Prodrug,** new extended-spectrum **triazole**
- Active against **yeasts, molds and dimorphic fungi**
- Approved for the treatment of:
  - **Invasive aspergillosis***
  - **Mucormycosis***
- Advantages include:
  - Availability of a water-soluble intravenous formulation
  - Excellent bioavailability of the oral formulation
  - Predictable pharmacokinetics
  - Devoid of nephrotoxicity
- **MOA:** Inhibits cytochrome P450 (CYP)–dependent 14α-lanosterol demethylation, which is essential for fungal cell membrane ergosterol synthesis.
- **Pharmacokinetics**
  - Metabolism: **Liver (CYP3A4/A5)**
  - Dose adjustment is not required in mild to moderate hepatic/renal impairment
- **Adverse effects**
  - Well tolerated
  - GIT: Nausea, vomiting, diarrhea
  - Rashes, headache
  - (↑) Hepatic enzyme levels
  - Infusion reactions (Chills, dyspnea, hypotension)

Ans: (b) Acts through blocking cytoplasmic proteins

Ref: *Miceli MH, Kauffman CA, Isavuconazole: A New Broad-Spectrum Triazole Antifungal Agent, Clin Inf Dis 2015;61:1558-1565*

16. Which of the following is relatively contraindicated in chronic kidney disease?

(a) Rivaroxaban (b) Apixaban
(c) Edoxaban (d) Dabigatran

Explanation:

Direct Oral Factor Xa Inhibitors include:

- Rivaroxaban
- Apixaban
- Edoxaban
- Dabigatran

Clinical Indications of Direct Oral Factor Xa Inhibitors

- Treatment of **acute venous thromboembolism**
- **Secondary** prevention of **venous thromboembolism**
- Prevention of **stroke** in **atrial fibrillation**
- **Thromboprophylaxis** after **hip or knee arthroplasty**

Use **of direct oral Factor Xa inhibitors in CKD and other co-morbid states**

- **Rivaroxaban**
  - Should be avoided in patients with **renal and hepatic dysfunction**
  - Use with caution in patients with **recent bleeding**
- **Apixaban**
  - Reduce the dose in patients with serum **creatinine ≥ 1.5 mg/dl, age >80 years** and weight <60 kg
  - Use with caution in patients with **recent bleeding**
- **Edoxaban**
  - Reduce the dose in patients with **CrCL 15-50 ml/min,** weight <60 kg and with concomitant potent P-glycoprotein inhibitor
  - Not recommended for patients with **CrCL < 15 ml/min**
  - Contraindicated if **CrCL > 95 ml/min**
  - Use with caution in patients with **recent bleeding**
- **Dabigatran**
  - Reduce the dose in patients with **CrCL 15-30 ml/min**
  - Not recommended for patients with **CrCL < 15 ml/min**

Ans: (b) Apixaban

Ref: *Hogg K, Weitz JL, A Blood Coagulation and Anticoagulant, Fibrinolytic and Antiplatelet Drugs, In: Brunton L, Chabner B, Knollman B Editors, Goodman and Gillman's The Pharmacological Basis of Therapeutics, 13th edition, New York: McGraw-Hill 2018, Page 601*

17. Erectile dysfunction (Hypogonadism) is caused by:

(a) Antihistamines (b) Leukotriene antagonists
(c) Thyroxine (d) Insulin glargine

Explanation:

- Drugs associated with erectile dysfunction:
  - **Antihypertensive drugs**
    - Beta blockers
    - Spironolactone
    - Thiazide diuretics
  - **Antiandrogens**
  - **LH releasing agonists and antagonists**
  - **CNS drugs**
    - Opioids
    - SSRIs
    - Benzodiazepines
    - Antipsychotics
    - TCAs
    - Phenytoin
  - **H_2 blockers**

Ans: (a) Antihistamines

Ref: *Yafi FA, Jenkins L, Albersen M, Corona G, Isidori AM, Goldfarb S et al., Erectile Dysfunction, Nat Rev Dis Primers 2017;2(1):1-47*

18. Prescription of PPIs can be done in all except:

(a) 40-year-old with Barret's espohagus
(b) 40-year-old with one episode of variceal bleeding
(c) 45-year-old with NSAID induced ulcer
(d) Stress ulcer in ICU patient

Explanation:

Proton Pump Inhibitors (PPIs):

- Include Esomeprazole, Lansoprazole, Omeprazole, Pantoprazole
- MOA: (-) of **H^+ K^+-ATPase pump**
- (↓) Daily production of acid (basal and stimulated) by 80%-95%

Clinical Indications of PPIs

- Gastroesophageal Reflux Disease (GERD)
- Erosive esophagitis
- Gastric ulcers
- Duodenal ulcers
- Helicobacter pylori eradication
- Zollinger-Ellison syndrome
- *Helicobacter pylori* eradication

Barret's Espohagus

- Replacement of normal esophageal cells with abnormal cells

- Associated with an increased risk of developing esophageal cancer
- Treatment depends upon the degree of cell dysplasia and regular follow up
- PPIs do not have any role in the management of Barret's espohagus

Ans: (a) 40-year-old with Barret's espohagus

Ref: *Sharkey KA, MacNaughton WK. A Pharmacotherapy for Gastric Acidity, Peptic Ulcers and Gastroesophageal Reflux Disease, In: Brunton L, Chabner B, Knollman B editors, Goodman and Gillman's The Pharmacological Basis of Therapeutics, 13th edition, New York: McGraw-Hill, 2018, Page 918*

19. Half-life of basiliximab is:

(a) 7 days (b) 7 hours
(c) 15 days (d) 24 hours

Explanation:

Basiliximab

- Chimeric mouse human monoclonal antibody against IL-2 receptor
- **$t_{1/2}$ =7 days**
- Indications
  - Prevention of **renal** and other **transplant rejection reaction**
- ADRs
  - Anaphylactic reactions
  - Opportunistic infections
- Other drug which acts as antagonist at **IL-2 receptor** is **daclizumab**

Ans: (a) 7 days

Ref: *Med Arh 2004;58(6): 373-76*

20. Colistin is not active against:

(a) *Pseudomonas aeruginosa* (b) *Serratia*
(c) *Klebsiella pneumoniae* (d) *Burkholderia*

Explanation:

COLISTIN

- **Polypeptide antibiotic**
- Has **low molecular weight**
- Produced by bacteria ***(Bacillus polymyxa*)***
- Used **topically** only due to its high systemic toxicity
- MOA:
  - Cause leakage from cell membranes
  - Bactericidal
- Antimicrobial spectrum:
  - Active against most **gram-negative microorganisms** except ***(Proteus, Serratia and Neisseria)***

- Exhibits synergistic activity with many other AMAs
- Resistance:
  - Resistance is never been a problem with this drug
  - No cross resistance with other AMAs
- ADRs:
- Topical application is associated with:
  - Well tolerated
  - Rashes
- Other polypeptide antibiotics include: Polymyxin-B, Bacitracin and Tyrothricin

Ans: (b) Serratia

Ref: *Tripathi KD, Essentials of Medical Pharmacology, 8th edition, New Delhi: Jaypee Brothers Medical Publishers, 2019, Page 809*

21. Regarding Artemisinin Pharmacokinetics all are true except:

(a) Dose adjustment not required in hepatic or renal failure (b) Has a long half life

(c) Oral bioavailability is around 30% (d) Autoinducers

Explanation:

Artemisinin and Its Derivatives

- Include **dihydroartemisinin, artemether** and **artesunate**
- Effective against severe *P. falciparum* malaria
- So far true resistance to these drugs have not been reported
- Pharmacokinetics
  - Oral bioavailability is **30%**
  - Peak serum concentration attains in 2-6 hours
  - Plasma protein binding ranges 43-82%
  - Plasma $t_{1/2}$ is **around 1-2 hours**
  - Marked inter individual variation in bioavailability through rectal administration
  - Autoinducers of CYP2B6 and CYP3A4 which can enhance their clearance by 5 folds

Ans: (b) Has a long half life

Ref: *Vinetz JM, Chemotherapy of Malaria, In: Brunton L, Chabner B, Knollman B editors, Goodman and Gillman's The Pharmacological Basis of Therapeutics, 13th Edition, New York: McGraw-Hill, 2018, Page 973*

22. A patient on Blinatumomab for refractory B cell ALL is now resistant to the drug. Which drug to be used?

(a) Vorinostat (b) Brentuximab

(c) Pembrolizumab (d) Tisagenlecleucel

Explanation:

Vorinostat

- Epigenetic modifying drug
- MOA: Histone Deacetylase inhibition
- Useful in relapsed/refractory ALL along with decitabine

Brentuximab

Pembrolizumab

Tisagenlecleucel

Ans: (d) Tisagenlecleucel

Ref: *Vairy S, Garcia JL, Teira P, Bittencourt H, CTL019 (tisagenlecleucel): CAR-T Therapy for Relapsed and Refractory B-Cell Acute Lymphoblastic Leukemia, Drug Design Dev Ther 2018;12:3885-3898*

23. Which of the following drugs is most useful for acute severe depression and has good side effect profile?

(a) RIMAs
(b) SSRIs
(c) Tricyclics
(d) MAO-inhibitors

Explanation:

SSRIs

- Selective Serotonin Reuptake Inhibitors (SSRIs) include fluoxetine, fluvoxamine, paroxetine, sertraline, citalopram, escitalopram

RIMAs

- Reversible Inhibitors of MAO–A (RIMAs) include moclobemide and clorgyline

Tricyclics

- Tricyclic Antidepressants (TCAs) include Imipramine, amitriptyline, trimipramine, clomipramine, desipramine, nortriptyline

SNRIs

- Serotonin and Noradrenaline Reuptake Inhibitors (SNRIs) include venlafaxine, duloxetine

Atypical Antidepressants

- Include trazodone, mirtazapine, bupropion, tianeptine, amineptine

Antidepressant drugs effective for acute severe depression include:

- TCAs
- SSRIs
- SNRIs
- Atypical antidepressants

ADRs of antidepressant drugs include:

- **TCAs**
  - Sedation, mental confusion
  - Anti-cholinergic
  - Cardiovascular (Hypotension and arrhythmias)

- Sexual dysfunction
- Hypersensitivity reactions
- Seizures

- **SSRIs**
    - Well tolerated, relatively safer with better acceptability
    - No anti-cholinergic effects
    - Little or no sedation
    - Devoid of α blocking action and hence no postural hypotension
    - Unlikely to produce arrhythmias or seizures

Ans: (b) SSRIs

Ref: *Tripathi KD, Essentials of Medical Pharmacology, 8th edition, New Delhi: Jaypee Brothers Medical Publishers, 2019, Page 491*

24. Which of the following drug do not act via NF-κβ:

(a) Sunitinib (b) Emetine

(c) Diltiazem (d) Bortezomib

Explanation:

- **Drugs which inhibits NF–κβ include:**
    - Bortezomib
    - Narasin
    - Bithionol
    - Sunitinib
    - Emetine
    - Fluorosalan
    - Lestaurtinib

Ans: (c) Diltiazem

Ref: *Biochem Pharmacol, 2010 May 1;79(9):1272-1280*

25. Which of the following is the most beta-1 selective antagonist?

(a) Acebutolol (b) Atenolol

(c) Metoprolol (d) Bisoprolol

Explanation:

Bisoprolol

- Highly selective **beta-1 selective antagonist** among the given drugs
- However **nebivolol** has **higher beta-1 selective** antagonist than **bisoprolol**
- **Beta-1 selective antagonist** include:
    - Acebutolol
    - Atenolol
    - Betaxolol

- Bisoprolol
- Celiprolol
- Esmolol
- Metoprolol
- Nebivolol

Ans. (d) Bisoprolol

Ref: *Goodman and Gillman's The Pharmacological Basis of Therapeutics, 2011, 12th edition, McGraw Hill, Burton LL, Page 328*

26. All are TNF alpha inhibitors except:

(a) Alemtuzumab
(b) Infliximab
(c) Adalimumab
(d) Eternercept

Explanation:

Alemtuzumab

- It is a humanized monoclonal antibody and has been approved for use in **chronic lymphocytic leukemia**
- It targets **CD52** which is expressed on **lymphocytes, monocytes, macrophages and natural killer cells**
- By targeting CD52, the drug causes **extensive lympholysis** by inducing **apoptosis of targeted cells**

Infliximab:

- It is a **chimeric anti-TNF-α** monoclonal antibody containing a **human constant region** and a **murine variable region**
- Binds with high affinity to **TNF-α** and prevents the **cytokine** from **binding to its receptors**

Adalimumab:

- It **recombinant human IgG monoclonal antibody** against **TNF-α** and given intravenously
- It is approved for use in the following conditions:
  - Rheumatoid arthritis
  - Ankylosing spondylitis
  - Crohn's disease
  - Juvenile idiopathic arthritis
  - Plaque psoriasis
  - Psoriatic arthritis.

Etanercept:

- It is not a **monoclonal antibody** but it targets **TNF-α**
- Contains the **ligand-binding portion** of a human TNF-α receptor fused to the Fc portion of human **IgG1,** and binds to **TNF-α** and prevents it from **interacting** with its **receptors**
- The following are its approved indications:
  - Rheumatoid arthritis
  - Ankylosing spondylitis
  - Plaque psoriasis

- Polyarticular juvenile idiopathic arthritis
- Psoriatic arthritis

Ans: (a) Alemtuzumab

Ref: *Goodman and Gillman's The Pharmacological Basis of Therapeutics, 12th edition, Page 1018*

27. Denosumab is used in:

(a) Osteomalacia (b) Osteoarthritis
(c) Osteoporosis (d) Osteosarcoma

Explanation:

Denosumab:

- RANKL binds to its cognate receptor RANK on the surface of precursor and mature osteoclasts, and stimulates these cells to mature and resorb bone
- **Osteoprotegerin (OPG),** which competes with RANK for binding to RANKL, is the physiological inhibitor of RANKL
- **Denosumab** is a human monoclonal antibody that binds with high affinity to **RANKL,** mimicking the effect of OPG, and thereby reducing the binding of RANKL to RANK
- Denosumab **blocks osteoclast formation** and **activation.** It increases **BMD** and **decreases bone turnover markers** when given subcutaneously once every 6 months
- **Indications:**
  - Prevention of skeletal-related events in patients with **bone metastases from solid tumors**
  - Treatment of adults and skeletally mature adolescents with **giant cell tumor of bone** that is unresectable or where surgical resection is likely to result in severe morbidity

Ans: (c) Osteoarthritis

Ref: *Goodman and Gillman's The Pharmacological Basis of Therapeutics, 12th edition, Page 1287*

PATHOLOGY

1. Examine this pedigree chart carefully. What type of transmission does it depict?

(a) AD inheritance
(b) AR inheritance
(c) X-linked recessive
(d) Holandric inheritance

Type of inheritance

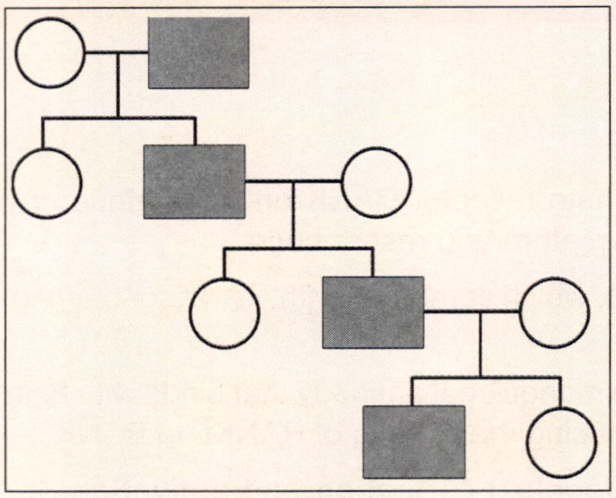

Explanation:

"Holandric" means, basically, a gene on the **Y chromosome** (in mammals) that does not have a homolog on the **X chromosome**

Holandric chromosome: Y-chromosome

- The differential region of Y-chromosome carries only Y-linked or holandric genes, **e.g., testis determining factor (TDF).** It is perhaps the smallest gene occupying only 14 pairs
- Other holandric genes are:
  - **Hypertrichosis** (excessive hairiness) **on pinna**
  - **Porcupine skin**
  - **Keratoderma dissipatum** (thickened skin of hands and feet); and
  - **Webbed toes**
- Holandric genes are directly inherited by a **son** from his **father**
- The pedigree shows **only men** are involved and **all the sons** of **affected dad are affected**

Ans: (d) Holandric inheritance

Ref: *Genetic Home Reference*

2. Interleukin involved in early phase of hematopoiesis is:

(a) IL–1
(b) IL–2
(c) IL–3
(d) IL–4

Explanation:

- **Interleukin** - 3 (IL–3) is a cytokine that regulates **hematopoiesis** by controlling the production, differentiation and function of **granulocytes and macrophages**

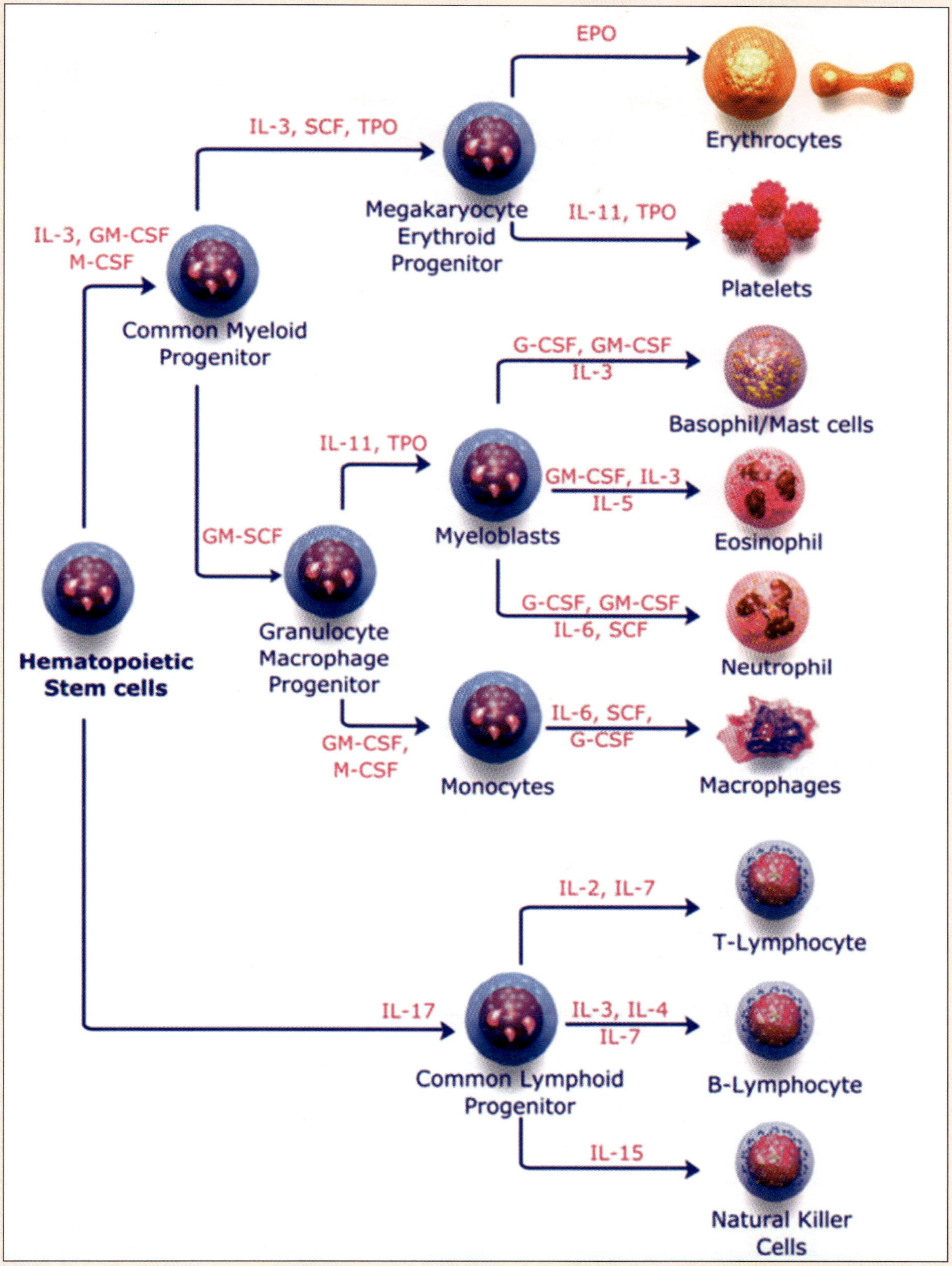

Ans: (c) IL–3

Ref: *Wintrobes Hematology, Chapter–Hematopoiesis*

3. A patient presents with bony pain. Investigations reveal ESR of 140 and Hb-6 gm. Peripheral smear (Figure) is shown. What type of chromosomal abnormality is most likely in this patient?

(a) t (14:16)
(b) t (6:14)
(c) Deletion 13
(d) t (11:14)

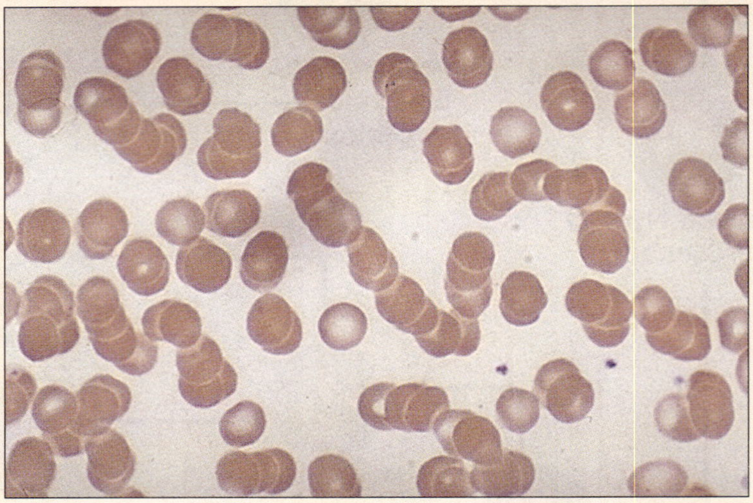

Explanation:

From the history, patient has

- Bone pain
- Elevated ESR (Due to IL6 in myeloma)
- Anemia
- Rouleaux formation

So the most compatible diagnosis with the available information is **Plasma cell Dyscrasia**

Myeloma and Genetics

- The most frequent chromosome translocations involve IGH on chromosome **14q32** and are present in 55-70% of PCMs
- Seven recurrent oncogenes are involved in 14q32 translocations: *CCND1* on 11q13 (involved in 16% of cases)

Molecular Prognostic factors. Few recalls say that it was about poor prognostic factors. (If then answer will be based on the below table)

Gene	Cytogenetic abnormality	Prognosis
FGFR3	T(4,14)	Poor
Cyclin D1	T(11,14)	Good
C-Maf	T(14,16)	Poor
13q (p53)	Loss of 13q14	Poor prognosis

- **Deletion of 13q14** carries poor prognosis*

Ans: (d) t (11:14)

Ref: *WHO, Hematology, Page 220-223*

4. A 15-year-old presents with a history of pain and swelling in the right thigh. Biopsy of the mass demonstrates osteosarcoma. His mother was diagnosed with breast cancer 1 year ago and his maternal grandmother died of breast cancer 10 years ago. The patient has three younger siblings. The siblings have an increased risk of developing which of the following cancers?

(a) Wilms
(b) Neuroblastoma
(c) Hepatoblastoma
(d) Glioma

Explanation:

- History is consistent with **Li Fraumeni Syndrome***

Diagnosis is Li Fraumeni Syndrome

A diagnosis of LFS and performing ***TP53* gene mutation** testing is considered for anyone with a personal and family history that meets 1 of the following 3 criteria:

Criterion 1
• A tumor belonging to the LFS tumor spectrum, before the **age of 46.** This means any of the following diseases: o **Soft-tissue sarcoma** o **Osteosarcoma** o **Pre-menopausal breast cancer** o **Brain tumor** o **Adrenal cortical carcinoma** o **Leukemia or** o **Lung cancer**
• At least 1 **first-degree or second-degree** family member with an **LFS-related tumor, except breast cancer** if the individual has breast cancer before the age of 56 or with multiple tumors
Criterion 2
• A person with **multiple tumors,** except **multiple breast tumors,** 2 of which belong to the LFS tumor spectrum and the first of which occurred before age 46
Criterion 3
• A person who is diagnosed with following regardless of family history. • **Adrenocortical carcinoma; or** • **Tumor** in the **choroid plexus,** a membrane surrounding the brain

Ans: (d) Glioma

Ref: *Genetic Home Reference*

5. Examine the peripheral smear (Figure) of a patient present with bony pain and bleeding. Which of the following will be the most probable diagnosis?

(a) CLL
(b) AML
(c) Myelofibrosis
(d) ALL

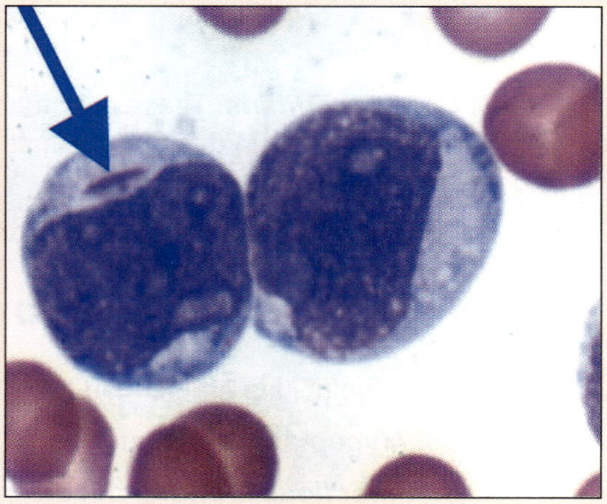

Explanation:

- **The Figure shows a cell with high N:C ratio and an Auer rod (blue arrow), diagnostic of Myeloblast**
- **Auer bodies** are rod-shaped crystalline inclusions formed of **azurophilic granules,** named after John Auer, though they were first recognized by Thomas McCrae
- Based on the electron microscopic finding way back in 1977, it was concluded that the formation of Auer rods is due to **defects** in the **formation, aggregation,** and concentration of the **peroxidase granules** in the **leukemic blasts**
- **Auer rods** are red staining, needle-like bodies seen in the cytoplasm of **myeloblasts,** and/or **progranulocytes** in certain leukemias
- **Auer rods are seen in:**
  - Acute myeloid leukemia
  - Acute promyelocytic leukemia
  - High-grade myelodysplastic syndromes
  - Myeloproliferative disorders
- Auer rods in neutrophils are a rare finding and their presence in neutrophils is suggestive of **nucleo-cytoplasmic asynchrony;** where the nuclear maturation has occurred, however, the cytoplasmic granule content is similar to that of immature myeloid cells

Ans: (b) AML

Ref: *WHO Hematology, Introduction to Myeloid Neoplasms*

6. Cold agglutinins are directly against which of the following RBC antigens?

(a) I (b) P
(c) Le (d) Rh

Explanation:

COLD AUTOANTIBODIES

- **Cold agglutinin – Anti I Antibody***
- **Cold Hemolysin type – Anti P Antibody***

Cold AIHA (Cold Agglutinin Type)

Cold antibody immunohemolytic anemia usually is caused by **low-affinity IgM antibodies** that bind to red cell membranes only at temperatures **below 30°C,** such as occur in **distal parts** of the body (e.g., ears, hands and toes) in **cold weather**

Mechanism:

- ***Cold agglutinins:*** These are monoclonal **IgM** antibodies that react at **4 to 6°C.** They are called agglutinins because the **IgM** directed against the **I antigen** present on the **RBCs** can agglutinate red cells due to its large size (pentamer)
- In addition IgM can **activate complement** resulting in the cells being coated with **C3b** followed by **extravascular hemolysis**

Examples:

- Cold agglutinins are seen in two clinical situations:
  - ***Mycoplasma*** pneumonitis*
  - ***Infectious mononucleosis****

- Vascular obstruction by the red cell agglutination can produce **Raynaud's pheonomenon,** which is characterized by ischemia in the fingers when expose to the cold
- More important, chronic forms of **cold agglutinin hemolytic anemia** occur in association with **certain B cell neoplasms** or as an idiopathic condition.

Ans: (a) I

Ref: *Robbins Pathology, 10th edition, Page 451*

7. Which of the following may show ABO incompatibility?

(a) Cryoprecipitate (b) Single Donor platelets
(c) Platelets rich platelets (d) FFP

Explanation:

Fresh Frozen Plasma (FFP)

- FFP is plasma prepared from **whole blood,** either from the primary centrifugation of whole blood into red cells and plasma or from a secondary centrifugation of platelet rich plasma
- The plasma is rapidly frozen to –25°C or colder within 8 hours of collection and contains normal plasma levels of stable clotting factors, albumin, immunoglobulin and Factor VIII at a level of at least 70% of normal fresh plasma

Unit of Issue:

- 200–300 ml.

Infection Risk:

- Capable of transmitting any agent present in cells or plasma which was undetected by routine screening TTIs, including HIV, hepatitis B and C, syphilis and malaria

Storage:

- FFP is stored at **–25°C** or colder for up to 1 year. Before use, it should be thawed in the blood transfusion centre between +30°C and +37°C.

Dosage: **15 ml/kg.**

Administration:

- Should be **ABO compatible**
- Infuse as soon as possible after thawing
- Labile coagulation factors rapidly degrade; use within 6 hours of thawing
- FFP may be beneficial if PT and/or partial thromboplastin time (PTT) >1.5 times normal
- FFP for volume expansion carries a risk of infectious disease transmission and other transfusion reactions (e.g., allergic) that can be avoided by using crystalloid or colloid solutions

Ans: (d) FFP

Ref: *WHO Manual of Blood Transfusion*

8. Juvenile myoclonic epilepsy is due to mutation in:

(a) GABRA 1 (b) CHRNA 2
(c) COL4A1 (d) FMRI

Explanation:

Juvenile Myoclonic Epilepsy Genes

- CACNB4
- CASR (Ca sensing receptor)
- GABRA1 (gamma-aminobutyric acid A receptor, alpha 1)
- GABRD (gamma-aminobutyric acid A receptor, delta) EFHC1

Ans: (a) GABRA 1

Ref: *Genetic Home Reference*

9. In alveolar variant of rhabdomyosarcoma, the resultant fusion protein is believed to function as:

(a) Activated growth factor receptor
(b) Chimeric transcription factor
(c) Constitutively active kinase
(d) Novel growth factor

Explanation:

Alveloar Variant of Rhabdomyosarcoma (ARMS)

- Subtype of the rhabdomyosarcoma soft tissue cancer family whose lineage is from **mesenchymal cells** and which is related to **skeletal muscle cells**
- Two fusion proteins can be associated with **alveolar rhabdomyosarcoma** (ARMS): ~60% of cases are positive for ***pax3-foxo1*** fusion gene, 20% **for *pax7-foxo1*** fusion gene, and 20% **are fusion negative** arms cases
- The translocations results in activation of the transcription factors which promote cell growth

Location: Soft tissue*, usually **Head and Neck*** regions

Origin: Precursor cells within muscle

Mx:

- Cells are often small with little cytoplasm
- Nuclei of the cells are round with normal, dull, chromatin structures
- Classical subtype: Nests of neoplastic cells arranged in alveolar spaces

Immunohistochemistry: Myogenin*, Myo D1*

Ans: (b) Chimeric transcription factor

Ref: *Sternberg Histopathology, Soft Tissue Tumors*

10. Most mature normoblast is:

(a) Orthochromic Normoblast
(b) Pronormoblast
(c) Polychromatic Normoblast
(d) Basophilic Normoblast

Explanation:

Order of Maturation is **Pronormoblast → Basophilic Normoblast → Polychromatic Normoblast → Orthochromic Normoblast (Also known as orthochromatic normoblast)***

Haematopoiesis:

- Physiologic process of blood cell formation
- Three stages of haematopoiesis include **mesoblastic stage (yolk sac), hepatic stage, and myeloid (bone marrow) stage**
- It takes place in **yolk sac and liver** in embryonic and early fetal life
- During embryonic and early foetal life, haematopoiesis occurs in the yolk sac (only erythoblasts) and the liver (all blood cells)
- It can also take place in **extramedullary sites** like spleen, lymph nodes and thymus.

Erythropoiesis: Is the physiologic process of red blood cell formation. Different stages of erythropoiesis are:

Morphology of each of the maturing erythroid cells

- **Pronormoblast (Proerythroblast):** 13–18 microns, round with thin rim of basophilic cytoplasm, large spherical nucleus with fine chromatin and 1–2 nucleoli
- **Basophilic (early) normoblast:** 12–17 microns; increase in deeply basophilic cytoplasm compared to pronormoblast and slightly smaller nucleus with slight chromatin condensation
- **Polychromatophilic (intermediate) normoblast:** 12–15 microns; round / ovoid with abundant, dull gray to gray green, variegated cytoplasm due to polyribosomes (basophilic) and hemoglobin (eosinophilic); round, condensed and basophilic nucleus has coarse granules that give it a cartwheel appearance
- **Orthochromatophilic (late) normoblast:** 8–12 microns; round / ovoid cells with pink orange uniformly staining cytoplasm, dark and opaque nucleus that may be pyknotic or in the process of being extruded
- **Reticulocyte:** 7–10 microns; cannot identify without **supravital stain (new methylene blue, brilliant cresyl blue)** that colors RNA deep blue and granular; must have at least 2 granules to classify as reticulocyte; cytoplasm is red to pale blue due to RNA, no nucleus is present; larger than mature erythrocyte and lacks central pallor, passes through the bone marrow sinus wall and endothelial cells into the circulating blood where it matures
- **Erythrocyte:** 7–8 microns; round / ovoid biconcave disc with orange red cytoplasm, no RNA, no nucleus; survives ~120 days in circulation

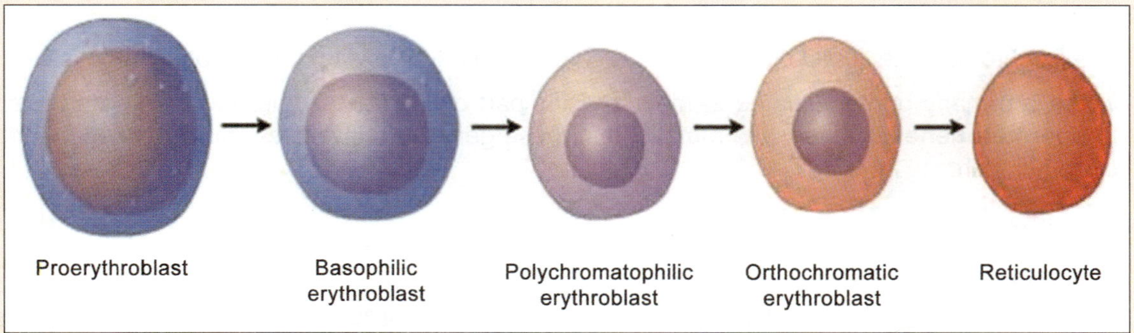

Figure: Morphology of maturing erythroid cells

ALSO NOTE:

Dyserythropoiesis

- Defective erythropoiesis.
- Microscopic features of dyserythropoies is seen in **normoblasts** are:
  - Inter-nuclear bridges
  - Nuclear budding
  - Karyorrhexis

- o Multinuclearity
- o Megaloblastoid features
- o Basophilic stippling
- o Howell-Jolly bodies
- o Cytoplasmic vacuolation
- o Ring sideroblast.

Ans: (a) Orthochromic Normoblast

Ref: *Tejindar Singh, 4th edition, Atlas and Text of Hematology, Volume I, Page 6 and Shirish M Kawthalkar, Essentials of Haematology, Page 3*

11. Examine this pedigree chart carefully. What type of transmission does this depict?

(a) Autosomal dominant (b) Autosomal recessive

(c) X-linked recessive (d) X-linked dominant

Type of inheritance

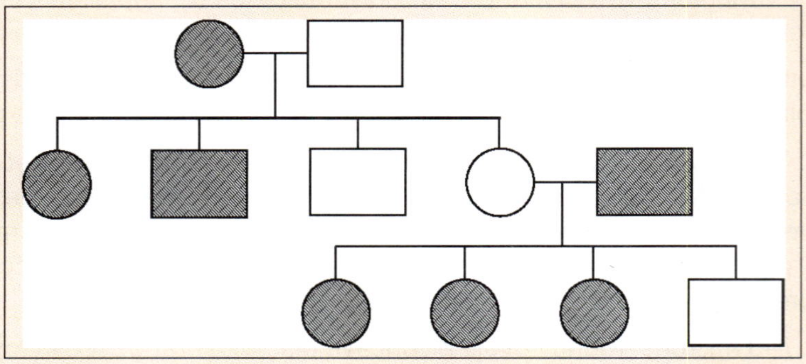

Explanation:

- All sex chromosome linked disorders are X-chromosome linked with majority being recessive
- There are many genes situated in male specific part of Y-chromosome and these are mostly related to **spermatogenesis.** Men with mutations in these genes are **infertile**. Thus, Y-linked inheritance are extremely rare.

X-linked Dominant Disorders

- Very rare
- These are transmitted by an **affected heterozygous female** to **50% of her sons** and **50% of her daughters**
- Affected father transmits to **all his daughters,** whereas the **sons** are **not affected** when the **mother is not affected**
- Example: **Vitamin D resistant rickets**

X-linked recessive disorders

- An **affected father does not** transmit the disorder to his **sons,** whereas all his **daughters are carriers**
- **Sons of heterozygous** mothers have **50% possibility** of inheriting the mutant gene
- Heterozygous / carrier females do not express complete phenotypic features of disorder
- As a result of **Lyon's hypothesis,** women have unpredictable cell proportion in which the mutant X-chromosome is active

X-linked recessive disorders:

System	Disease
Musculoskeletal	Duchenne muscular dystrophy
Blood	• Hemophilia A and B • Chronic granulomatous disease • Glucose-6-phosphate dehydrogenase deficiency
Immune system	• Agammaglobulinemia • Wiskott-Aldrich syndrome
Metabolic diseases	• Diabetes insipidus • Lesch-Nyhan syndrome
Nervous system	• Fragile X syndrome

Ans: (d) X-linked dominant

Ref: *Robbins and Cotran Pathologic Basis of Disease, 9th edition, Page 142*

12. Formula for calculationg Reticulocyte production index:

(a) Retic × hct/ normal hct
(b) Corrected ret × hct /45 | maturation index
(c) Reticulocyte percentage × RBC count
(d) Reticulocyte counted × 100/ number of red cells

Explanation:

- **Reticulocytes** are **immature red blood cells** containing remnants of **ribosomal RNA***
- They can be demonstrated using supravital stains like **New methylene blue*** and **brilliant cresyl blue***
- **Reticulocyte count:** Is determined by counting **reticulocytes among 1000 RBCs** and is expressed as **percentage**
  - This parameter is used to **assess the erythropoiesis of bone marrow**
  - The normal reticulocyte count in **adults** is **0.5-2.5%** and in **newborns** is **2-5%**
- **Corrected retiulocyte count:** Is the reticulocyte count corrected for **degree of anaemia**
- **Absolute reticulocyte count:** Is total number of **reticulocytes in 1 cmm of blood**
  - Normal absolute reticulocyte count is **50,000-1,00,000/cmm**

Reticulocyte Production Index:

- Reticulocytes after formation spend **2 days in bone marrow** and a **day in peripheral** blood to become a mature red cell
- There is **compensatory premature release** of reticulocytes in severe **haemolytic** anaemia and **acute blood loss**
- Thus, these reticulocytes need **extra time for maturation**
- In such circumstances, in order to avoid undue overestimation of daily reticulocyte production, **reticulocyte production index** is derived using the formula **ret* hct /45 | maturation index**
- Maturation index according to PCV are:
  - PCV >35% : 1
  - PCV 25-35% : 1.5
  - PCV 15-25% : 2
  - PCV 5-15% : 2.5

(**Note:** A value of 45 is considered as normal hematocrit)

Causes of reticulocytosis	Causes of reticulocytopaenia
• Acute blood loss • Haemolytic anaemia • Response to therapy in nutritional anaemias	• **Deficient red cell production** o Iron deficiency anaemia o Anaemia of chronic disease o Aplastic anaemia • **Anaemia due to marrow infiltration:** o Leukaemia o Lymphoma o Metastatic cancer • **Ineffective erythropoiesis:** o Megaloblastic anaemia

Ans: (b) Corrected ret* hct /45 | maturation index

Ref: *Dr.Tejindar Singh, 4th edition, Atlas and Text of Hematology, Volume I, Page 7; Shirish M Kawthalkar, Essentials of Haematology, Page 63*

13. Which of the following is involved in apoptosis pathway?

(a) myc
(b) p53 and caspases
(c) APC
(d) VHL

Explanation:

Apoptosis

- Defined as 'coordinated and internally programmed cell death'.
- It has a role both in physiologic and pathologic conditions.

Apoptosis in Physiologic Processes:

- **Embryo development**
- **Hormone dependent involution** of cells like **breast** after lactation, **endometrial shedding**
- Replacement following cell destruction in intestine
- **Thymus involution**

Apoptosis in Pathologic Processes:

- **Tumor cell death** exposed to chemotherapeutic drugs
- **Cell death** in **graft versus host disease*** and **graft rejections***
- CD 4+ T cells depletion in **AIDS**
- Cell death in viral infections, **e.g., Councilman bodies**
- Atrophy of organs and tissues on withdrawal of stimuli, e.g., **prostatic atrophy** following **orchiectomy**
- **Neurodegenerative diseases:** Alzheimer's disease, Parkinson's disease
- **Acute myocardial infarction**

Morphologic Features:

- **Cell shrinkage**
- Chromatin condensation
- Formation of cytoplasmic blebs and apoptotic bodies

- Phagocytosis of apoptotic cells or cell bodies

Mechanisms:

- Apoptosis results from activation of enzymes called **caspases** which are **cysteine proteases** that cleave proteins after **aspartic residues**
- Two phases of apoptosis are:
  - **Initiation** phases and
  - **Execution** phases
- Two pathways in initiation phase that activate **caspase:**
  - ***Intrinsic (mitochondrial) pathway***
  - ***Extrinsic (death receptor) pathway***

Intrinsic (Mitochondrial) Pathway:

- Results from increase in **mitochondrial permeability** and release of **cytochrome C**
- **Antiapoptotic genes: BCL2, BCL-XL, and MCL1***
- **Pro-apoptotic genes: BAX and BAK***
- **Sensors: BAD, BIM, BID, Puma and Noxa***
- **Cytochrome C** binds to **APAF-1** resulting in formation of **apoptosome** which activates **caspase-9**

Extrinsic (Death Receptor) Pathway:

- Activation of death receptors present on plasma membrane of wide variety of cells
- Cell death receptors: **TNF-1, Fas (CD 95)***
- Ligands: **FasL**
- **Fas and FasL** bind resulting in activation of **FADD,** which further activates **caspase-8 and 10**
- Inhibitor: **FLIP**

Execution Phase:

- Executioner caspases–**Caspase-3 and 6***
- Activate DNAase leading to DNA cleavage
- The formation of **apoptotic bodies** is followed by **phagocytosis**

Note:

- **Necroptosis–**A programmed form of necrosis, or inflammatory cell death–caspase independent
- **Pyroptosis–**Another type of programmed cell death which is associated with release of IL-1 which produces fever

Ans: (b) p53 and caspases

Ref: *Robbins and Cotran Pathologic Basis of Disease, 9th edition, Page 52*

14. Russell's Bodies are found in:

(a) Neutrophils (b) Basophils
(c) Mott cells (d) Mast cells

Explanation:

Russell Bodies:

- Large, homogeneous, **eosinophilic immunoglobulin** containing inclusions
- Seen in **Plasma cells** synthesising **excess** of **immunoglobulins**
- Named after a Scottish physician, William Russell
- They represent **distended endoplasmic reticulum***
- These are result of insufficient transport of protein within cell
- They are not tissue specific
- They are **periodic acid Schiff positive***
- Immunohistochemistry: positive for **CD 38, CD138, CD79a, kappa and lambda**
- Russell bodies containing plasma cells are **autofluorescent***
- Conditions where Russell bodies are seen:
    - **Chronic inflammation**
    - **Plasma cell**
- Plasma cell containing aggregates of Russell bodies is called as **Mott cells***

Also Note: Other cells/bodies seen in myeloma

- **Flame cells:** Myeloma cells having orange-red colored periphery
- **Dutcher bodies:** Intranuclear inclusions
- **Pseudo-Gaucher cells**

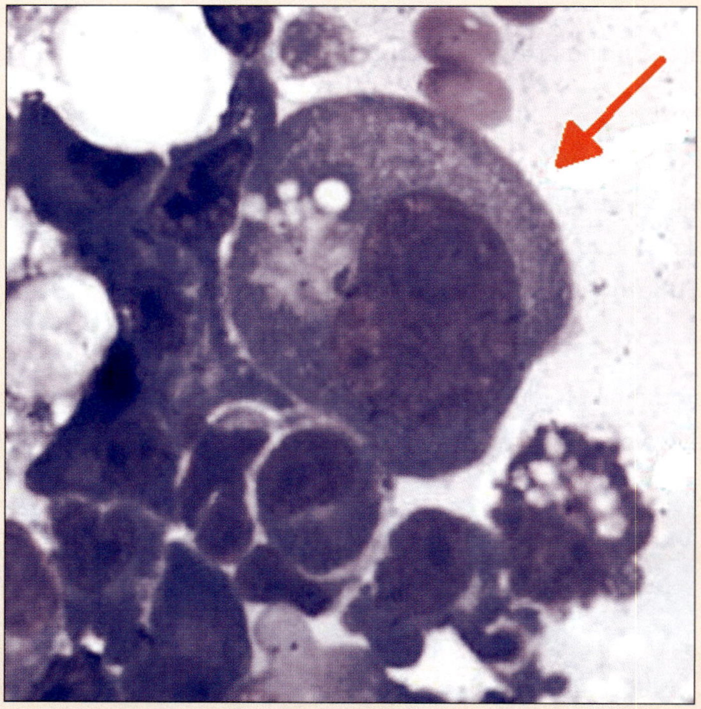

Figure: Mott cell with Russel bodies (Red arrow)

Ans: (c) Mott cell

Ref: *Robbins and Cotran Pathologic Basis of Disease, 9th edition, Page 601*

15. All are poor prognostic markers of Multiple myeloma except:

(a) t (1:14) (b) t (14:16)

(c) 1q gain (d) t (14:20)

Explanation:

PLASMA CELL MYELOMA

- Multifocal neoplastic proliferation of plasma cells, associated with M protein in serum and/or urine and oragan damage
- The two most important **poor prognostic factors** are:
  - **β2–macroglobulin***
  - **Deletion of 13q14. t(4;14)***
- **t (11;14)* has good prognosis**
- Conventional prognostic factors are: Ki- 67, plasma cell mass, anaemia, hypercalcemia, raised creatinine levels, hypoalbuminemia.

International Myeloma Working Group Criteria for multiple myeloma are:
Clonal plasmacytosis ≥ 10% on bone marrow biopsy with one or more of following myeloma defining events:

- **End-organ damage:**
  - Hypercalcaemia: Serum calcium > 0.25 mmol/L
  - Renal insufficiency: Creatinine clearance < 40 ml/minute or serum creatinine > 177 µmol/L (> 2 mg/dL)
  - Anaemia: A haemoglobin value < 100 g/L
  - Bone lesions: One or more osteolytic lesion on skeletal radiography, CT, or PET/CT
- **Any one of the following biomarkers of malignancy:**
  - Clonal bone marrow plasma cell percentage > 10%
  - Involved: Uninvolved serum free light chain ratio >100
  - > 1 focal lesion on MRI

Smouldering (asymptomatic) myeloma:

- Bone marrow plasma cells are clonal and 10-60%
- M protein > 8 g/dl without myeloma defining event

MAYO STRATIFICATION OF MYELOMA

- **Standard risk**
  - t(11; 14)
  - t(6; 14)
  - Hyperdiploidy
- **Intermediate risk**
  - t(4; 14)
  - Del 13
  - Hypodiploidy
- **High risk**
  - Del 17p

- t (14:16)
- t (14:20)

Non-secretory myeloma:

- Accounts for 1% of myeloma
- **M protein** is **absent** on serum and urine immunofixation
- Pathogenesis: Impaired secretion of immunoglobulin by neoplastic plasma cells

Ans: (a) t (1: 14)

Ref: *WHO Classification of Tumors of Haematopoietic and Lymphoid Tissue, 2017, Page 243*

16. Examine the gross kidney image. What is the diagnosis?

(a) Granular contracted kidney
(b) Flea bitten kidney
(c) Spongy kidney
(d) Hemorrhagic kidney

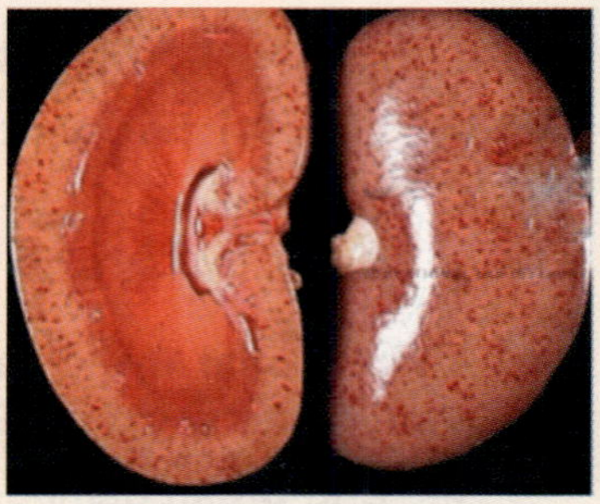

Explanation:

Flea Bitten Kidney:

- Enlarged edematous kidney with petechial haemorrhages and microinfarctions on renal cortical surface
- It is due to thromboses in arcuate and interlobular arteries
- **Causes:**
  - **Acute post streptococcal glomerulonephritis***
  - **Malignant hypertension***
  - **Infective endocarditis***
  - Wegener's granulomatosis
  - Rapidly progressive glomerulonephritis
  - **Type IV SLE***
  - Leptospirosis
  - Polyarteritis nodosa
  - Leukemia

Granular Contracted Kidney:

- Bilateral, symmetrical, small and contracted kidney with diffusely granular cortical surface
- Capsule is adherent at places
- Cortex in atrophic on cut section
- **Cause: Chronic glomerulonephritis**

Ans: (b) Flea bitten kidney

Ref: *Robbins and Cotran Pathologic Basis of Disease, 9th edition, Page 912*

17. Examine the renal histopathology slide. What is the probable diagnosis?

(a) Membranoproliferative GN
(b) Rapidly proliferative GN
(c) PSGN
(d) Diabetic nephropathy

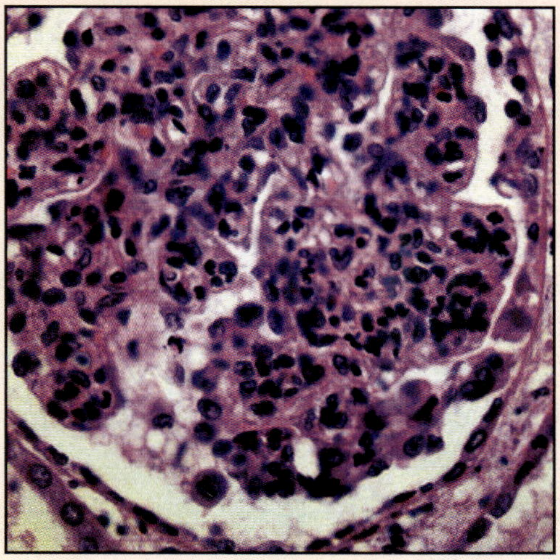

Explanation:

- HPE shows diffuse involvement of **glomeruli,** Enlarged hypercellular glomeruli and Acute proliferative lesions s/o **Acute infectious GN**

Post Streptococcal GN:

- Common in developing countries
- Commonly affects children between 2 and 14 years
- Rare in adults more than 40 years accounting for 10%
- It follows 1-2 weeks of streptococcal pharyngitis and impetigo
- Nephritogenic strains implicated in etiology of PSGN are **types 12, 4 and 1**
- Titres of antibodies that are raised are: **ASLO, anti-DNAse B, anti-streptokinase, anti-NADase, anti-hyaluronidase**
- Hypocomplementemia seen
- Gross: **Flea bitten kidney**
- **Microscopy:**
  - Diffuse involvement of glomeruli
  - Enlarged hypercellular glomeruli
  - Acute proliferative lesions
- **EM findings:** Electron dense irregular deposits on epithelial side glomerular basement membrane (humps)
- **IF: IgG and C3 along GBM**
- **Clinical Features:**
  - Microscopic or intermittent haematuria
  - **Red cell casts**
  - Mild non-selective proteinuria (less than 3 gm per 24 hours)
  - Hypertension
  - Periorbital oedema
  - Oliguria

Ans: (c) Post streptococcal GN

Ref: Robbins and Cotran Pathologic Basis of Disease, 9th edition, Page 909

18. NKX3-1 immunohistochemical used for diagnosis of:

(a) Colorectal carcinoma
(b) Pancreatic carcinoma
(c) Prostate
(d) Renal cell carcinoma

Explanation:

- **NKX3.1** is transcription factor protein and plays a pivotal role in normal development of prostate
- Human NKX3.1 gene is present on **chromosome 8p21** and it undergoes loss of heterozygosity during progression of prostate malignancy
- It is expressed specifically in **prostate gland**
- Its expression is **androgen dependent** and is lost/**reduced in prostate malignancy**
- It increases p53 stability and activity
- It is highly restricted to prostate epithelial cells and thus serves as a diagnostic **biomarker for tumors originating from prostate**
- It is more **sensitive and specific** than PSA and PSAP
- It can act as transcriptional activator or repressor
- NKX3.1 loss is an initiating event in PIN
- Loss of expression of NKX3.1 is significantly associated with hormone refractory disease and metastasis
- Location on IHC–nucleus
- Normally highly expressed in prostate and at lesser level in testis, salivary gland, bronchial submucosal glands, transitional epithelium of ureter
- Positive staining is seen in primary and metastatic **carcinoma of prostate, invasive lobular and ductal carcinoma of breast, ovary and endometrium**

Ans: (c) Prostate

Ref: *Robbins and Cotran Pathologic Basis of Disease, 9th edition, Page 1209*

19. A 5-year-old boy came with c/o Cervical lymphadenopathy. Microscopic picture of lymph node biopsy show Starry sky app. Which of the following translocation is unlikely to be seen in this condition?

(a) t (2, 8)
(b) t (8, 22)
(c) t (8, 14)
(d) t (11, 18)

Explanation:

Burkitt lymphoma (BL) is an aggressive lymphoma than can present at extranodal sites or as acute leukemia. It is characterized by monotonous medium sized B cells with deeply basophilic cytoplasm and abundant mitotic figures

Types:

- African (endemic) Burkitt lymphoma
- Sporadic (nonendemic) Burkitt lymphoma
- Associated with HIV

Pathogenesis:

- All forms are linked with translocations of **MYC gene** on chromosome 8
- MYC is a transcriptional regulator
- Molecular trait of BL is translocation of **MYC** at band **8q24** to the IGH region on chromosome **14q32, t(8;14),** or less commonly to the IGK locus on **2p12 [t(2;8)]** or the IGL locus on **22q11 [t(8;22)]**

Invariably **endemic BLs are infected with EBV** latently. EBV is associated with 25% of HIV associated BL and 15 to 20% of sporadic BL.

Morphology:

- Diffuse infiltration of 10-25 µm lymphoid cells with round to oval nuclei, coarse nuclei and abundant basophilic cytoplasm
- **High mitotic index**
- Numerous **apoptotic cells** seen
- Tumor cells consist of many lipid vacuoles in cytoplasm–**Starry sky pattern***

Burkitt-like lymphoma with 11 q aberration: Is a type of lymphoma that is similar to BL morphologically, but lack rearrangements involving MYC. Alternativey, they have alterations of chromosome 11q.

Also Note:

- **t (11, 18)** is associated with **mucosa-associated lymphoid tissue (MALT) type lymphoma**

Ans: (d) t (11, 18)

Ref: *Dr. Tejindar Singh, 4th edition, Atlas and Text of Hematology, Volume I, Page 443; WHO Classification of Tumors of Hematopoietic and Lymphoid Tissues 2017, Page 330; Robbins and Cotran Pathologic Basis of Disease. Robbins and Cotran Pathologic Basis of Disease, 10th edition, Page 591*

20. 4-year-old boy presenting with Cryptorchidism, short stature and on auscultation, harsh ejection systolic murmur is heard in pulmonary area. What is the hematological abnormality found in this condition?

(a) Transient Myeloproliferative disorder
(b) Juvenile Myelomelanocytic leukemia
(c) Pseudo Pelger Huetanomaly
(d) Burkitt lymphoma

Explanation:

- Clinical history is consistent with Noonan's syndrome

JUVENILE MYELOMELANOCYTIC LEUKEMIA (JMML)

- **JMML** is **BCR/ABL negative** entity which is regarded as **MDS/MPN** syndrome seen in children aged **4 years or less**
- It is an aggressive disease characterized by proliferation of granulocytic and monocytic series.

Association: Neurofibromatosis type I and Noonan's syndrome.

Clinical Features:

- Hepatosplenomegaly
- Lymphadenopathy
- Non-specific symptoms–Pallor, fever, infection, bleeding, cough, poor weight gain, a maculopapular rash
- Those with **NF I:** café-au-lait spots, neurofibromas, glioma, freckles, Lisch nodules

- With **Noonan's syndrome:** Congenital heart defects, specifically, pulmonary stenosis, cryptorchid testis, low hair line, wide set eyes, low set ears, delay in learning

DIAGNOSTIC CRITERIA

I. Clinical and hematologic features (all 4 features mandatory)
- Peripheral blood monocyte count 1 x 10^9/L
- Blast percentage in PB and BM < 20%
- Splenomegaly
- **Absence of Philadelphia chromosome** (BCR/ABL 1 rearrangement)

II. Genetic studies (1 finding sufficient)
- Somatic mutation in PTPN11 or KRAS or NRA5
- Clinical diagnosis of NFI or NF1 mutation
- Germ line CBL mutation and loss of heterozygosity of CBL

III. For patients without genetic features, besides the clinical and hematologic features listed under I, the following criteria must be fulfilled; Monosomy 7 or any other chromosomal abnormality or at least 2 of the following criteria:
- **Hemoglobin F** increased for age
- Myeloid or erythroid precursors on PB smear
- GM-CSF hypersensitivity in colony assay
- Hyperphosphorylation of STAT5

Differentials:
- Viral infections: Like herpes virus, EBV, CMV
- Acute myelomonocytic leukemia
- CML
- Osteopetrosis

Transient Myeloproliferative Disorder:
- Associated with Down's syndrome
- It develops in utero and is usually diagnosed prenatally or within 3 months of birth and then it resolves spontaneously
- Approximately 10% with TMD **develop acute megakaryoblastic leukemia**
- It is characterised by proliferation of non-malignant mekaryoblast
- **GATA1 mutations** are seen in few
- **Bleeding tendency** is the common manifestation

Ans: (b) Juvenile myelomonocytic leukemia

Ref: *WHO Classification of Tumors of Hematopoietic and Lymphoid Tissues 2017, Page 89*

21. Investigation to distinguish hemophilia A and lupus anticoagulant:

(a) Factor 8 assay (b) dRVVT
(c) Vwf assay (d) Aptt

Explanation:

ANTIPHOSPHOLIPID SYNDROME (APS)

- Previously called **lupus anticoagulant syndrome** is an acquired autoimmune syndrome
- Characterised by **thromobosis, repeated miscarriages and thrombocytopenia**
- Presence of antiphospholipid antibodies **(aPL)** (like lupus anticoagulant–LA), anticardiolipin antibodies **(aCL)** or antibodies directed against different proteins, mainly beta 2-glycoprotein I **(β_2GPI)**

Incidence: 1-2% in general population. Four times more common in **females** with mean age being 32 years

Clinical Features:

- The common manisfestation of APS is **deep vein thrombosis** and **arterial thrombotic** manifestations are mostly in the form of **cerebrovascular accidents**
- The common obstetric complications include repeated **fetal losses, pre-eclampsia and premature births**
- Other clinical manifestations include **livido reticularis** and thrombocytopenia
- Antiphospholipid antibodies are IgG, IgA or IgM antibodies that bind to phospholipid. β_2GPI is the most important antigenic target of aPL
- Moreover, it seems that only aPL with high affinity for β_2GPI are pathologically relevant
- **Val 247 allele** may be one of the genetic risk factors for development of APS

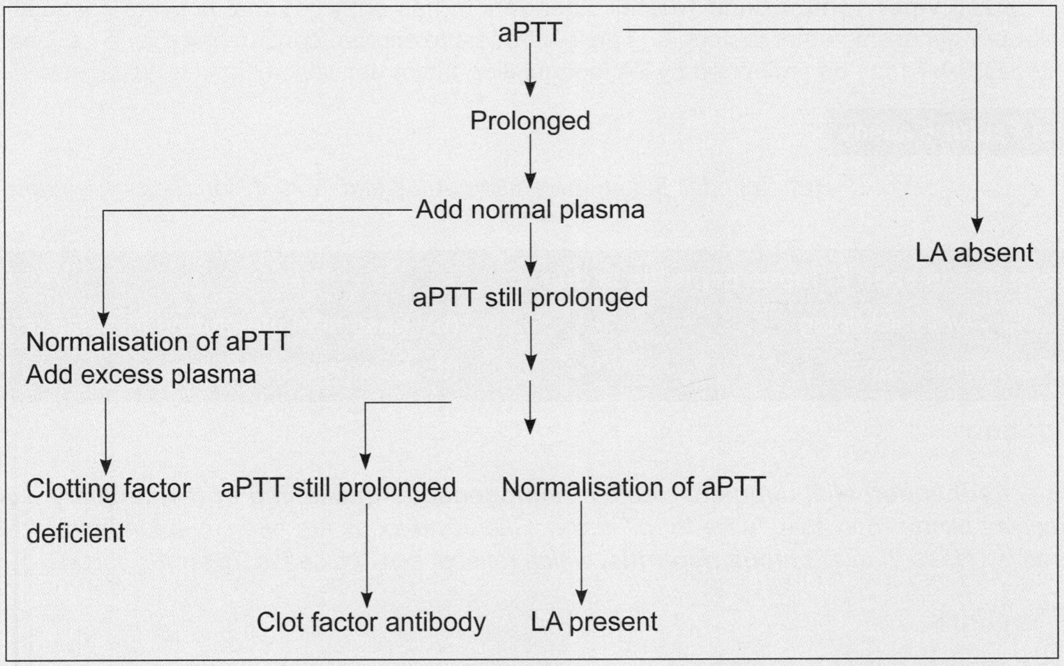

REVISED CRITERIA FOR APS (SAPPORO)

A. Clinical Criteria

1. **Vascular Thrombosis:** ≥ 1 clinical episode of arterial/venous/small thrombosis without presence of inflammation of vessel wall confirmed by imaging/histopathology
2. **Pregnancy Morbidity**
   (a) ≥ 1 unexplained death of a morphologically normal (on Ultrasound or direct examination of fetus) fetus 10 weeks gestation
   (b) ≥ 1 premature birth of a morphologically normal neonate ≤ 34th week because of pre-eclampsia, eclampsia or placental sufficiency
   (c) ≥ 3 unexplained consecutive spontaneous abortions < 10th week of gestation

B. Lab Criteria–All lab criteria should be present in 2 or

>2 occasions at least 12 weeks apart using recommended proceedings

1. **aCL anticardiolipin antibody** IgG/IgM +ve on ≥ 2 occasions at least 6 weeks apart, tested by ELISA and present in medium or high titre
2. **Lupus anticoagulant** positive on at least 2 occasions, at least 6 weeks apart as per the guidelines of International society of thrombosis and hemostasis
   (a) Prolonged phopholipid dependent coagulation, e.g., APTT, KCT (Kaolin clotting lime), dilute Russel Viper Venom time
   (b) Failure to correct the above test by mixing with normal platelet poor plasma
   (c) Correction of the time with addition of excess phospholipid
   (d) Exclusion of other coagulopathies
3. **Anti-β2-GPI antibody**–IgG/IgM isotope present in titre > 99th percentile measured by standardised procedure – ELISA

Catastrophic APS: Life threatening severe thrombotic microangiopathy resulting in multi organ failure. Seen in <1% of APS patients

APS nephropathy: Triad of focal cortical atrophy, fibrous intimal hyperplasia of renal vessels and thrombotic microangiopathy

Dilute Russell viper venom time: Russell viper venom has enzymes that activate coagulation factors V and X directly bypassing other factors. It is an in vitro test to screen, confirm or exclude LA insensitive APTT reagents). DRVVT may be prolonged by LA, coagulation factor deficiencies and anticoagulants.

Ans: (a) Factor 8 assay

Ref: *Tejindar Singh, 4th edition, Atlas and Text of Hematology, Volume I, Page 586*

22. Wire loop lesion seen in lupus nephritis is due to:

(a) Capillary wall thickening
(b) Basement membrane thickening
(c) Subepithelial deposits
(d) Sclerosis of mesangium

Explanation:

"Prominent ***subendothelial deposits*** *create a* ***homogeneous thickening of the capillary wall,*** *which are seen by light microscopy as a* ***"wire-loop"*** *lesion. Such wire loops are often found in both focal and diffuse proliferative* ***(class III or IV) lupus nephritis,*** *which reflects active disease." (Ref: Robbins)*

Lupus Nephritis

- Lupus nephritis results from the deposition of circulating immune complexes, which activate the complement cascade leading to ***complement-mediated damage, leukocyte infiltration,*** activation of ***procoagulant factors,*** and release of various ***cytokines***
- The presence of antiphospholipid antibodies trigger a ***thrombotic microangiopathy***
- The most common clinical sign of renal disease is **proteinuria**, but **hematuria, hypertension,** varying degrees of **renal failure,** and active **urine sediment** with **red blood cell casts** can also be present
- **Anti-dsDNA antibodies** that fix complement correlate best with the presence of renal disease
- **Hypocomplementemia** is common in patients with acute lupus nephritis **(70–90%)**
- **Class I** nephritis describes ***normal glomerular histology*** by any technique or normal light microscopy with minimal mesangial deposits on immunofluorescent or electron microscopy

- **Class II** designates mesangial immune complexes with ***mesangial proliferation.*** Both class I and II lesions are typically associated with minimal renal manifestation and normal renal function
- **Class III** describes ***focal lesions*** with proliferation or scarring, often involving only a segment of the glomerulus
- **Class IV**–Global, diffuse proliferative lesions. ***Most common type–Worst Renal prognosis***
- The **class V** lesion describes ***subepithelial immune deposits*** producing a ***membranous*** pattern

Classification for Lupus Nephritis

Class I	**Minimal mesangial**	**Normal histology with mesangial deposits**
Class II	**Mesangial proliferation**	Mesangial hypercellularity with expansion of the mesangial matrix
Class III	**Focal nephritis**	Focal endocapillary ± extracapillary proliferation with focal subendothelial immune deposits and mild mesangial expansion
Class IV	**Diffuse nephritis**	Diffuse endocapillary ± extracapillary proliferation with diffuse subendothelial immune deposits and mesangial alterations
Class V	**Membranous nephritis**	Thickened basement membranes with diffuse subepithelial immune deposits; may occur with class III or IV lesions and is sometimes called mixed membranous and proliferative nephritis
Class VI	**Sclerotic nephritis**	Global sclerosis of nearly all glomerular capillaries

Ans: (a) Capillary wall thickening

Ref: *Robbins Pathologic Basis of Disease, 9th edition*

23. CGG repeat sequence is found in:

(a) Fragile X syndrome
(b) Huntington's chorea
(c) Dentatorubropallidolusyian atrophy
(d) Machado Joseph disease

Explanation:

Expansions affecting non-coding regions

Disease	Protein	Repeating Sequence
Fragile X syndrome	FMR-1 protein	**CGG***
Friedrich ataxia	Frataxin	**GAA***
Myotonic dystrophy	Myotonic dystrophy protein kinase (MDPK)	**CTG***

Expansions non-coding regions

Disease	Protein	Repeating Sequence
Spinobulbar muscular atrophy (Kennedy Disease)	Androgen Receptor	CAG
Huntington Disease	Huntington	CAG
Dentatorubral-pallidoluysian atrophy (Haw River Syndrome)	Atrophin–1	CAG
Spinocerebellar ataxia type 1	Ataxin–1	CAG
Spinocerebellar ataxia type 2	Ataxin–2	CAG
Spinocerebellar ataxia type 3 (Machado Joseph Disease)	Ataxin–3	CAG

Contd.

Contd.

Spinocerebellar ataxia type 6	Alpha 1a–Voltage-dependent calcium channel subunit	CAG
Spinocerebellar ataxia type 7	Ataxin–7	CAG

Ans: (a) Fragile X syndrome

Ref: *Robbins and Cotran, Pathologic Basis of Disease, 8th edition, Elsevier, 2011, Page 168*

24. Which of the following is secreted by TH-1 helper cells?

(a) IL-1 (b) IL-2

(c) IL-4 (d) IL-3

Explanation:

- **Type 1 T helper (Th1)** cells produce:
  - ***Interferon-gamma***
  - ***Interleukin (IL)-2***
  - ***Tumour necrosis factor (TNF)-beta***
- These factors activate macrophages and are responsible for:
  - **Cell-mediated immunity**
  - **Phagocyte-dependent protective responses**
- **CD4 cells (T helper cells)** on **activation** leads to one of the three well defined subsets **TH1, TH2 and TH17 subset**

Subset	TH1	TH2	TH17
Cytokine produced	• IFN-gamma • IL-12 • IL2	• IL-4 • IL-5 • IL-13	• IL-17 • IL-22 • Chemokines
Immunological reactions triggered	• Macrophage activation • Stimulation of IgG antibody production	• Stimulation of IgE production • Activation of mast cells and eosinophils	• Recruitment of neutrophils • Monocytes
Host Defense against	• Intracellular microbes	• Helminthic parasites	• Extracellular bacteria • Fungi
Role in Disease	• Immune-mediated chronic inflammatory diseases (often autoimmune)	• Allergies	• Immune-mediated chronic inflammatory diseases (often autoimmune)

EXTRA EDGE:

Two transcription factors have been found that play a critical role in the choice between becoming a **Th1 or a Th2 cell.**

- **T-bet** for Th1 cells
- **GATA3** for Th2 cells

Ans: (b) IL-2

Ref: *Robbins Pathology, 9th edition, Page 107*

25. Which is not a feature of Lofgren syndrome?

(a) Uveitis
(b) Erythema nodosum
(c) Polyarthralgia
(d) Bilateral hilar adenopathy

Explanation:

Lofgren Syndrome:

- Lofgren's syndrome is an acute form of sarcoidosis
- Triad comprises:
  - **Erythema nodosum**
  - **Bilateral hilar lymphadenopathy (BHL)**
  - **Polyarthralgia or polyarthritis**
- Associated with HLA-DQB1 and HLA-DRB1
- **Uveitis** and **elevated levels of ACE,** are often **absent** in patients with Lofgren's syndrome (eye involvement, 5%; elevated ACE levels, 50%)
- Lofgren's syndrome was regarded as a **self-limiting disease** that is generally resolved within the first year

Ans: (a) Uveitis

Ref: *Robbins Pathology, 9th edition*

MICROBIOLOGY

1. Autoinfection is NOT seen in:

(a) *H. nana*
(b) *H. diminuta*
(c) Strongyloidosis
(d) *Taenia solium*

Explanation:

- What is **AUTO-INFECTION?**
  - The infection of a primary host with a parasite, especially a helminth, in such a way that the complete life cycle of the parasite happens in a single host, without the involvement of another host.
- For example, Autoinfection in **Enterobius vermicularis*** occur by finger contamination with the eggs from the perineal skin or faeces and by gravid segments reaching the stomach by retrograde peristalsis from jejunum

Parasites causing AUTOINFECTION (Mnemonic: HETS-C^2):

- ***H**ymenolepis nana*
- ***E**nterobius vermicularis*
- ***T**aenia solium*
- ***S**trongyloides stercoralis*
- ***C**ryptosporidium parvum*
- ***C**apillaria philippinensis*

Ans: (b) *H. diminuta*

Ref: *Paniker's Textbook of Parasitology, 6th edition, Page 149-151*

2. Smallest helminth among the following is:

(a) *Hymenolepis diminuta*
(b) *Hymenolepis nana*
(c) *Diphyllobothrium latum*
(d) *Balantidium coli*

Explanation:

Smallest and Largest Parasites

Parasite classification	Smallest parasite	Largest parasite
Protozoa	*Dientamoeba fragilis*	*Balantidium coli*
Cestode	*Hymenolepsis nana*	*Diphyllobothrium latum*
Trematode	*Heterophyes heterophyes*	*Fasciolopsis buski*
Nematode	*Trichinella spiralis*	*Ascaris lumbricoides*

Note:

- Balantidium coli is NOT an helminth, it is a protozoan.
- Helminths include Cestode, Trematode and Nematodes.

Ans: (b) *Hymenolepis nana*

Ref: *KD Chatterjee 13th edition, Page 138-140, 147-150, 168*

3. Tungiasis is:

(a) Ecto parasite skin infection
(b) Ecto parasite intestinal infection
(c) Endo parasite skin infection
(d) Endo parasite intestinal infection

Explanation:

Tungiasis

- **Inflammatory skin disease** caused by infection with the female ectoparasitic ***Tunga penetrans*** (also known as **chigoe flea, jigger, nigua or sand flea**), found in the tropical parts of Africa, the Caribbean, Central and South America and India.
- ***Tunga penetrans*** (“***foot bug***”**)** is the smallest known flea, measuring **1 mm** across.
- The impregnated female burrows into the skin of the feet of mammals, preferring humans and pigs, where they cause a mother of pearl-coloured papule with a central dark punctum, produced by the enlarging flea abdomen which extrudes a large number of eggs. The female flea dies and is sloughed from the skin.
- It causes **skin inflammation**, severe **pain**, **itching**, and a lesion at the site of infection that is characterized by a **black dot at the center of a swollen red lesion**, surrounded by what looks like a **white halo**.
- Desquamation of the skin is always seen, especially after the flea expands during hypertrophy.

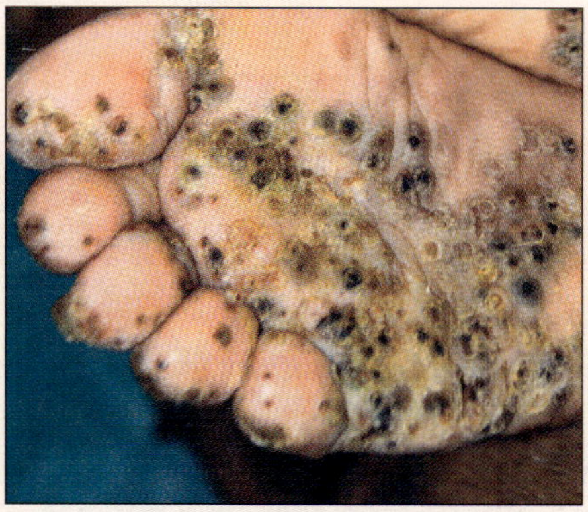

Figure: Tungiasis of soles

Ans: (a) Ecto parasite skin infection

Ref: *Clinical Infectious Diseases, 2nd edition, David Scholossberg, Page 167*

4. Gold standard investigation for Zika virus:

(a) PCR
(b) Plaque reduction neutralization test
(c) IgM antibodies
(d) RT-PCR

Explanation:

- **Nucleic acid amplification test (NAAT)**, is a generic term referring to all molecular tests used to detect viral genomic material.
- **NAAT assays** are the preferred method of diagnosis because they can provide confirmed evidence of infection.
- Despite the specificity of molecular testing, **false positive NAAT results** have been reported in rare cases and may depend on the type of NAAT assay performed and patient population (i.e., limited or no prevalence of viral transmission) being tested.
- This problem can be exacerbated when Zika virus testing is performed on patient populations not recommended in the Zika testing algorithms.

- Due to the temporal nature of Zika virus RNA in serum and urine, a negative NAAT does not exclude recent Zika infection.
- For this reason, **Zika virus immunoglobulin (Ig) M antibody testing** is recommended in certain situations. IgM levels are variable, but generally become positive starting in the **first week** after onset of symptoms and continuing for up **to 12 weeks** post symptom onset or exposure, but may **persist for months to years**.
- Zika virus antibody testing is also complicated by **cross-reactivity** with other **flaviviruses**, which may make conclusive determination of which flavivirus is responsible for the person's recent infection difficult.
- With IgM antibody testing, false-positive results are more common than with NAAT and can occur due to non-specific reactivity or cross-reactivity with other flaviviruses.
- **Plaque reduction neutralization tests (PRNT)** are quantitative assays that measure virus-specific neutralizing antibody titers. PRNTs can resolve false-positive IgM antibody results caused by non-specific reactivity and at times help identify the infecting virus.
- Molecular diagnostics-based on **RT-PCR** is highly **specific and sensitive**, and considered the **"gold standard" for ZIKA Virus detection**. RT-PCR is effective in **serum, semen and saliva within <14 days post infection**, and possibly much longer in **urine and semen.**

Ans: (d) RT-PCR

Ref: https://www.cdc.gov/zika/laboratories/types-of-tests.html

5. Gene responsible for semisynthetic penicillin resistance in Methicillin resistant Staph aureus (MRSA):

(a) Mec A (b) Mec B

(c) Mec D (d) Mec C

Explanation:

- The **mecA gene** allows a bacterium to be resistant to antibiotics such as **methicillin, penicillin** and **other penicillin-like antibiotics**.
- The most commonly known carrier of the **mecA gene** is the bacterium known as **MRSA**. Apart from staphylococcus aureus and other Staphylococcus species, it can also be found in **Streptococcus pneumoniae** strains resistant to penicillin-like antibiotics. In staphylococcus species, **mecA** is spread on the SCCmec genetic element.
- **SCCmec or staphylococcal cassette chromosome *mec***, is a mobile genetic element of staphylococcal bacterial species.
- This genetic sequence includes the *mecA* gene coding for resistance to the **antibiotic methicillin** and is the only known way for staphylococcus strains to spread the gene in the wild by **horizontal gene transfer**.
- The emergence of methicillin-resistant staphylococcal lineages is due to the **acquisition and insertion of the SCC*mec* element** into the chromosome of susceptible strains.
- SCC*mec* elements are highly diverse in their structural organization and genetic content and have been classified into types and subtypes.
- Till date, **eight SCC*mec* types** have been described for ***Staphylococcus aureus***. The first three SCC*mec* elements were designated as **types I, II and III**.
- These were followed by reports of SCC*mec* **types IV to VIII**. Recently, MRSA infections have increasingly been reported among groups of patients with no apparent connection to hospitals.
- The **community acquired MRSA (CA-MRSA) strains** that cause non hospital-associated infections are characteristically susceptible to many antibiotics, **harbour type IV SCCmec**, which is much smaller in size than other SCC*mec* elements, and contains no other antibiotic resistance genes except *mec*A.
- **In contrast to CA-MRSA**, the majorities of health care-associated MRSA (HCA-MRSA) strains carry one of two types of SCC*mec*, **type II or III**, and show characteristics of **multidrug resistance**.

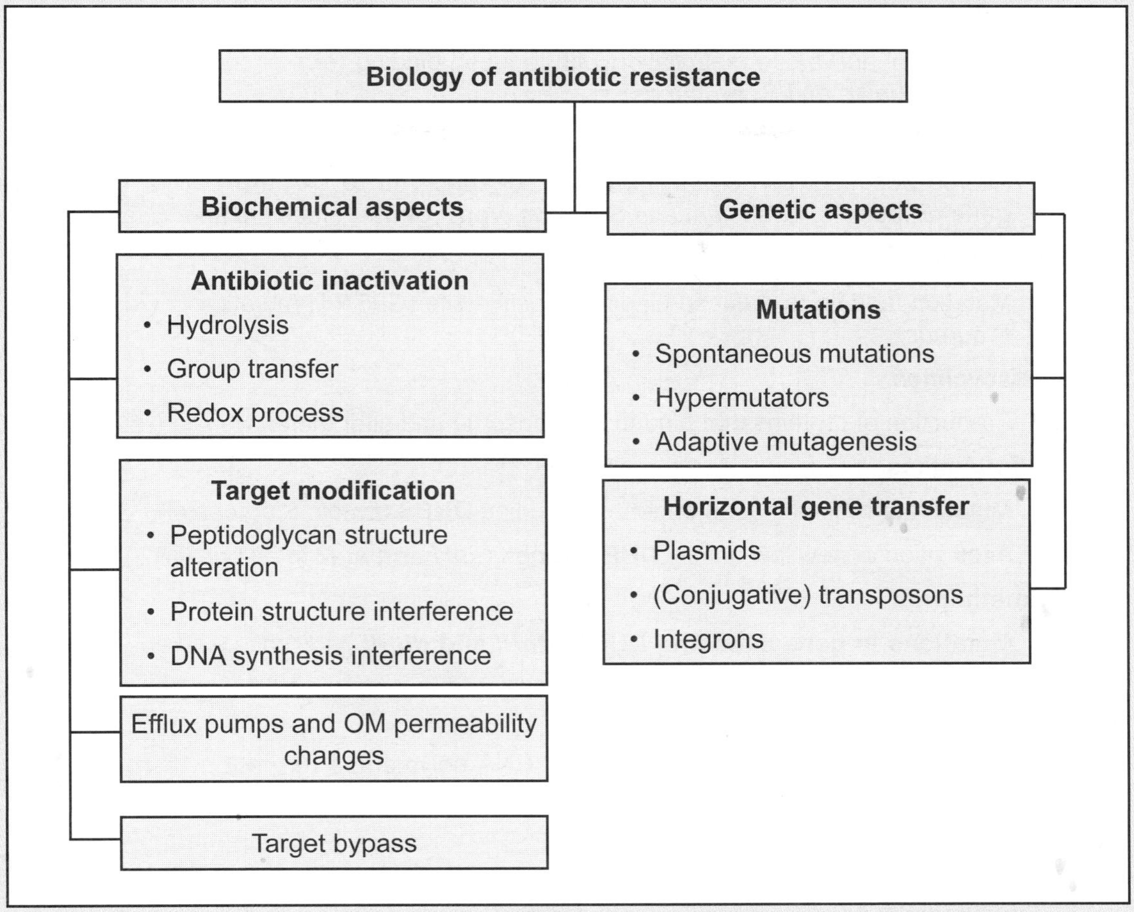

EXTRA EDGE:

Mechanism of Drug Resistance*:

(A) ***Resistance by efflux mechanism:***

- Quinolones–NorA in *S.aureus*
- Chloramphenicol–*cmlA* and *flo*-encoded efflux in *E.coli and Salmonella spp*.
- Macrolides–*mef*-encoded efflux in *S.pneumoniae and S. pyogenes*
- Tetracyclines–*tet* genes encoding efflux proteins in GPB and GNB

(B) ***Resistance by Decreased uptake:***

- **Aminoglycosides**
  - Changes in outer membrane permeability–*P.aeruginosa*
  - Altered electrical potential (AEP)–Bacterial respiration generates AEP (inhibits movements aminoglycosides across cell membrane–anaerobes and facultative anaerobes, e.g, *Enterococci*)

(C) ***Resistance by Altered target mutation:***

- **β-Lactams–Altered PBP(s)**
  - **PBP 2a** (***mec*A** in *S.aureus* and CONS)
  - **PBP 2x, PBP 2b, PBP 1a** (acquired from other Streptococci by transformation *S.pneumoniae)*
  - **PBP 5** (point mutation)–*E.faecium*
- **Quinolones**
  - Mutation leading to reduced binding to active sites (***gyr*A** in enteric GNB and *S.aureus*, ***gyr*A and *par*C** in *S.pneumoniae)*

- **Macrolides**
  - Ribosomal active site methylation with reduced binding (*erm*-encoded methylases in *S.aureus, S.pneumoniae and S. pyogenes)*
- **Glycopeptides**
  - Altered peptidoglycan cross link target (**D-Ala-D-Ala to D-Ala-D-Lac or D-Ala-D-Ser**; **Van A gene**–*E.faecalis, E.faecium and S.aureus,* **VanB gene**–*E.faecium and E.faecalis)*
- **Oxazolidinones**
  - Mutation leading to reduced binding to active site (G2576U mutation in rRNA in *E.faecium and S.aureus)*
- **Tetracyclines**
  - Production of proteins that bind to the ribosome and alter the active site (***tet*(M)** in GPB)
- **Sulfonamides**
  - Mutation or recombination of genes encoding **DHPS** (*E.coli, S.aureus and S.pneumoniae)*
  - Acquisition of new low affinity **DHPS genes (*sul1* and *sul2*** in enteric GNB)
- **Trimethoprim**
  - **Mutations in gene encoding DHFR** (***dhfrI* and *dhfrII*** in *E.coli, S.aureus, S.pneumoniae and H.influenzae)*
- **Rifampin**
  - Mutation leading to reduced binding to RNA polymerase (**Mutation in *rpoB*** in *S.aureus and M.tuberculosis)*

Ans: (a) Mec A

Ref: *Ananthanarayan and Paniker, 9th edition, Page 201-204; Jawetz's Microbiology; Harrison's Infectious Disease, 2nd edition, Page 406, 430, 500 and Manual of Clinical Microbiology. In Versalovic J,10th edition, Washington DC; ASM Press 2011: Vol 1, 1093*

6. Panton-Valentine leukocidin is produced by:

(a) *Staphylococcus epidermidis*
(b) Pseudomonas
(c) *Vibrio cholerae*
(d) *Staphylococcus aureus*

Explanation:

Virulence factors produced by *Staphylococcus aureus*:

- Slide coagulase positive due to Clumping factor
- Tube coagulase positive
- Panton valentine Leukocidin – Furunculosis and MRSA infection
- Bicomponent toxin – Leukocidin and γ hemolysin (Synergohymenotropic toxin)
- Anti teichoic acid Abs – Found in patients with S.aureus endocarditis
- Fibrinolysin (**Staphylokinase**) – Spread of infection

Toxins of *Staphylococcus aureus*

(A) Cytolytic Toxins:

- α **Hemolysin**–Most important hemolysin
  - Protein inactivated at 70°C, but reactivated paradoxically at 100°C.

- Lyses rabbit erythrocyte but is less active against human erythrocytes.
- Leucocidal, cytotoxic, dermonecrotic, neurotoxic and lethal.

- β **Hemolysin** – Shows 'hot cold phenomenon'. Sphingomyelinase, hemolytic for sheep cells.
- γ **Hemolysin** – Bi component protein.
- δ **Hemolysin** – Detergent like effect on cell membranes.
- **Leucocidin** (**Panton valentine Toxin**) – Bi component toxin associated with furunculosis.
- **Synergohymenotropic toxin**: Bi component toxin such as Leucocidin and γ Hemolysin.

(B) Enterotoxin: (A, B, C1-3, D, E and H):

- Preformed, heat stable toxin, responsible for staphylococcal food poisoning which occur 2-6 hours after consuming meat and fish, milk or milk products.
- Source – Usually food handler which is carrier.
- Mechanism – Toxin acts directly on autonomic nervous system (Vagal stimulation) and vomiting centre.
- Type A toxin is responsible for most cases.

(C) Toxic shock syndrome toxin (TSST):

- Toxic shock syndrome is multisystem disease presenting with fever, hypotension, myalgia, vomiting, diarrhea, mucosal hyperemia, erythematous sunburn, rash, disorientation or altered consciousness seen mostly in menstruating women using highly absorbent vaginal tampons.
- **TSST-1 = Enterotoxin F = Pyrogenic Exotoxin C** is responsible for most cases.
- Vomiting is due to direct stimulation of ANS rather than local action.
- Staph. Enterotoxin and TSST are **super antigen** leading to an excessive and non-regulated immune response.

(D) Exfoliative/Epidermatolytic Toxin/ET/Exfoliation:

- Cause **staphylococcal scalded skin syndrome (SSS).**
- Severe form is called **Ritter's disease** in neonate and toxic epidermal necrolysis in elderly.
- Milder form are **pemphigus neonatorum** and **bullous impetigo**.
- There are two types: ETA and ETB, toxin possess serine protease activity which triggers exfoliation.

Ans: (d) *Staphylococcus aureus*

Ref: *Ananthanarayan and Paniker, 9th edition, Page 201-203*

7. Which of the following is an amplifying host for Japanese encephalitis?

(a) Pig (b) Herons

(c) Horse (d) Egrets

Explanation:

JAPANESE ENCEPHALITIS

- *Vector:* – **Culex tritaneorhynchus** (most important)
  - C. vishnvi
  - C. gelidus.
- Man is an **incidental** '**dead end**' host.
- **Animal host :**

- o **Pigs** – Major vertebrate host.
  - – Not manifest any symptoms so acts as an **amplifiers**.
- o **Cattles and buffaloes** – Act as **mosquito attractants**.
- o **Horses** – Only domestic animals which shows signs of **encephalitis**.
- o **Birds host** – **Pond herons** (reservoir host), Cattle egrets, poultry and ducks.

- Incubation period in man – **5-15 days**.
- No viremia in cattle and horse.
- Average period between onset of illness and death is about **9 days.**

Please remember: In Japanese encephalitis

- **Reservoir host**: Herons and Egrets, ducks, pigeons, sparrows (Rarely)
- **Amplifier host:** Pigs
- **Vector transmitting:** Culex tritaeniorhynchus
- **Accidental host:** Human, cattle and horse

Ans: (a) Pig

Ref: *Ananthanarayan and Paniker, 9th edition, Page 521-523*

8. Trans ovarian transmission is seen among:

(a) *Rickettsia akari* (b) *Rickettsia rickettsii*

(c) *Rickettsia prowazekii* (d) *Rickettsia typhi*

Explanation:

- **Transovarial or transovarian transmission** occurs in certain arthropod vectors as they transmit pathogens from parent arthropod to offspring arthropod. For example, Rickettsia rickettsii, carried within ticks, is passed on from parent to offspring tick by transovarial transmission.
- Rickettsial infections transmitted by **TICKS*** have trans ovarian transmission among them to act as vectors as well as reservoirs.

Rickettsial diseases

Group	Species	Disease	Vector
Typhus fever	*R. prowazekii*	Epidemic typhus and Brill Zinsser	Louse
	R. typhi	Endemic typhus	Flea
Spotted fever	*R. rickettsii*	Rocky mountain spotted fever	**Tick**
	R.conori	Indian tick typhus	**Tick**
	R. akari	Rickettsial pox	Mite (Gamasid)
Scrub typhus	*O.tsutsugamushi*	Scrub typhus	Mite (Trombiculid)

ALSO NOTE:

- **Scrub typhus**, caused by **O. tsutsugamushi,** transmitted by **trombiculid mite** also shows **transovarian spread*.**

Ans: (b) Rickettsia rickettsii

Ref: *Ananthanarayan and Paniker, 9th edition, Page 406-408*

9. A retroviral positive patient presents with frequent diarrheal episodes. Stool examination reveals acid-fast oocyst of size 8-10 microns. What could be the probable diagnosis?

(a) *Toxoplasma gondii* (b) *Cryptosporidium parvum*

(c) *Coccidioides immitis* (d) Sarcocystis

Explanation:

CRYPTOSPORIDIUM PARVUM

- Cryptosporidia were first observed in the gastric mucosal crypts of laboratory mice by Tyzzer in 1907. Its importance as a pathogen causing diarrhea in animals was recognized in 1971 and the first case of human infection reported in 1976.
- Cryptosporidium has assumed great importance as a frequent cause of intractable diarrhea in **AIDS patients.**
- Natural infection with C.parvum is present in many species of **birds** such as chicken, turkey, and of animals including cattle, sheep, goats and cats.
- The oocysts of Cryptosporidium in stool samples are modified **acid fast** (cold Ziehl-Neelsen) stain positive, measuring about **6-10 μm.**

AIDS RELATED DIARRHEA

- The most common infectious organisms causing AIDS-related diarrhea include:
  - Cytomegalovirus (CMV)
  - Cryptosporidium parvum
  - Microsporidia
  - Isospora belli
  - Giardia lamblia
  - Mycobacterium avium-intracellulare (MAC)

Acid fast structures:

- *Cryptosporidium parvum*
- *Legionella micdadei*
- *Mycobacterium tuberculosis*
- *Lepra bacilli*
- Atypical mycobacteria
- Sperm head
- Egg of *Taenia saginata*
- *Cyclospora cayetanensis*
- *Isospora belli*
- *Nocardia spp*
- *Rhodococcus spp*
- Bacterial spores
- Egg of Schistosoma hematobium
- Hooklet of hydatid cyst
- Leptomonad promastigote

Ans: (b) *Cryptosporidium parvum*

Ref: *KD Chatterjee, 13th edition, Page 52-63*

10. Encrusted cystitis is caused by:

(a) *Corynebacterium xerosis*
(b) *Corynebacterium urealyticum*
(c) *Corynebacterium renale*
(d) *Corynebacterium pseudotuberculosis*

Explanation:

- **Encrusted cystitis (EC) is** a rare condition defined by **bladder mucosal struvite calcifications**.
- First reported in 1914, EC is caused by urea-splitting bacteria, often ***Corynebacterium urealyticum****
- This member of skin flora is present in 12% of the population. It is slow-growing and is often missed on rapid urine culturing.
- EC is generally preceded by **urologic instrumentation**.
- Treatment involves **glycopeptides antibiotics, urine acidification**, and **removal of calcifications**. Corynebacterium can form biofilms and may persist if calcifications are not completely removed.

Ans: (b) *Corynebacterium urealyticum*

Ref: *https://www.ncbi.nlm.nih.gov/pmc/articles/PMC3294293/ ; Ananthanarayan and Paniker, 9th edition, Page 242*

11. Elek's gel precipitation test used for diagnosing:

(a) *Corynebacterium jakeium*
(b) *Corynebacterium diphtheriae*
(c) *Clostridium tetani*
(d) *Clostridium perfringens*

Explanation:

Corynebacterium diphtheriae:

General characteristics	Cultural characteristics
• **Babes-Ernst/Volutin/Metachromatic granules**, gram positive bacilli • **Chinese letter or cuneiform arrangement**	• Selective media **– Hoyle's potassium tellurite blood agar**/Tinsdale media • Enriched media–**Loeffler's serum slope**
Virulence factors	**Clinical features**
• DT coded by **corynephages** • Toxin for Diphtheria toxin – **Park William Strain 8**	• Types of Diphtheria – Faucial, Respiratory, Cutaneous and invasive form • **Most common diphtheria** – Respiratory form • Diphtheria is toxaemia not bacteremia– **Cardiotoxicity** • **Pseudo membrane formation**–Leathery • **Bull neck appearance** of lymph nodes
Diagnosis	**Treatment**
• **Albert/Neisser's/Ponders staining** • **Toxigenic test**–In vivo: **Guinea pig inoculation** and in vitro: **Elek's gel precipitation** test, Immunochromatographic strip test • Test for immune status – **Schick test** • Matrix assisted laser desorption/ionization time of light (MALDI-TOF) and PCR	• Main stay of treatment – **Diphtheria Antitoxin** • DOC – **Erythromycin or Procaine Penicillin G** • **Active immunization** by diphtheria toxoid

Ans: (b) *Corynebacterium diphtheriae*

Ref: *Ananthanarayan and Paniker, 9th edition, Page 240*

12. Which among the following is a Coccobacilli is:

(a) *Escherichia coli* (b) *Listeria monocytogenes*

(c) *Haemophilus influenzae* (d) *Pseudomonas aeruginosa*

Explanation:

- A **coccobacillus** (plural **coccobacilli**) is a type of bacterium with a shape intermediate between **cocci** (spherical bacteria) and **bacilli** (rod-shaped bacteria). Coccobacilli are very short rods which may be mistaken for cocci.
    - ***Haemophilus influenzae, Gardnerella vaginalis***, and ***Chlamydia trachomatis*** are coccobacilli.
    - ***Aggregatibacter actinomycetemcomitans*** is a Gram-negative coccobacillus prevalent in subgingival plaques.
    - ***Acinetobacter strains*** may grow on solid media as coccobacilli.
    - ***Bordetella pertussis*** is a Gram-negative coccobacillus responsible for causing whooping cough. ***Yersinia pestis***, the bacteria that causes plague, is also coccobacillus.
    - ***Coxiella burnetti*** is also a coccobacillus.
    - Bacteria from the genus ***Brucella*** are medically important coccobacilli that cause brucellosis.
    - ***Haemophilus ducreyi***, another medically important Gram-negative coccobacillus, is observed in sexually transmitted disease, chancroid.

Ans: (c) *Haemophilus influenzae*

Ref: *Ananthanarayan and Paniker, 9th edition*

13. All are true about Immune reconstitution inflammatory syndrome (IRIS) except:

(a) It occurs when CD4 cell count is less than 50

(b) Develops after initiation of anti-retroviral therapy

(c) Associated with delayed type of hypersensitivity

(d) Does not require specific antimicrobial therapy for recovery

Explanation:

IMMUNE RECONSTITUTION INFLAMMATORY SYNDROME (IRIS)

- Immune reconstitution inflammatory syndrome (IRIS) is a condition seen in some cases of AIDS or immunosuppression, in which the immune system begins to recover, but then responds to a previously acquired opportunistic infection with an overwhelming inflammatory response that paradoxically makes the symptoms of infection worse.

DIAGNOSTIC CRITERIA

- **Major criteria**
    1. Atypical presentation of "opportunistic infections (OI) or tumours" in patients responding to antiretroviral therapy.
    2. Decrease in plasma HIV RNA level by at least 1 $\log_{10}$ copies/mL.
- **Minor criteria**
    1. Increased blood CD4+ T-cell count after HAART.

2. Increase in immune response specific to the relevant pathogen, e.g., DTH response to mycobacterial antigens.
3. Spontaneous resolution of disease without specific antimicrobial therapy or tumour chemotherapy with continuation of antiretroviral therapy.

Ans: (a) It occurs when CD4 cell count is less than 50

Ref: *https://www.ncbi.nlm.nih.gov/pmc/articles/PMC3221202/*

14. Which among the following is bile esculin positive and shows growth in 6.5% sodium chloride?

(a) *Streptococcus agalactiae* (b) *Streptococcus pneumoniae*
(c) *Enterococcus faecalis* (d) *Streptococcus viridans*

Explanation:

Species or common name	Lancefield group	Hemolysis	Laboratory test	Common diseases caused
S. pyogenes	A	Beta	Bacitracin sensitive; PYR test positive; Ribose not fermented	Upper respiratory tract infections; Pyoderma; Rheumatic fever; Glomerulonephritis
S. agalactiae	B	Beta	CAMP test, hippurate hydrolysis	Neonatal meningitis; Septicemia
S. equisimilis	C	Beta	Ribose and trehalose fermentation	Pharyngitis, Endocarditis
S. angiosus	A,C,F,G, Untypable	Beta (alpha, gamma)	Group A strains bacitracin resistant, PYR negative	Pyogenic infections
Enterococcus spp. ***(E. faecalis, E. faecium and E.durans)***	D	Gamma (alpha, beta)	Growth in 6.5% NaCl; PYR positive	Urinary tract infections, Endocarditis, Suppurative infections
Nonenterococcal group D species (*S. bovis, S. equinus*)	D	Gamma	No growth in 6.5% NaCl.	Endocarditis
Viridans streptococci	Not typed	Alpha (gamma)	Optochin resistant	Endocarditis (***S. sanguis***); Dental caries (***S. mutans***)

Enterococci diagnosis:

- Non hemolytic gram positive cocci, **may show α, β, γ hemolysis** in rabbit and horse blood
- Grows in the presence of **6.5% NaCl and 40% bile**
- **PYR +ve**
- **Bile esculin** hydrolysis positive
- Resistant to penicillin and low level aminoglycosides
- Vancomycin resistant enterococci mediated by **Van gene**
- ***E. faecium*** – 80% resistant to vancomycin
- ***E. faecalis*** – 7% resistant to vancomycin

Ans: (c) *Enterococcus faecalis*

Ref: *Ananthanarayan and Paniker, 9th edition, Page 230-234*

15. All the following mycobacteria produces pigment except:

(a) M. kansasii (b) M. simiae

(c) M. avium (d) M. scrofulaceum

Explanation:

Classification of Atypical Mycobacteria (Runyons classification)

Atypical mycobacteria/Non-tuberculous mycobacteria/Mycobacteria Other than Tubercle bacilli

- **Group I – Photochromogens**
  - Produce pigment when exposed to light but not in dark
  - E.g. *M marinum, M simiae, M kansasii*
- **Group II – Scotochromogens**
  - Form pigment even in dark
  - E.g. *M scrofulaceum, M gordonae*
- **Group III – Non-photochromogens**
  - Do not form pigment even on exposure to light
  - Eg. *M avium, M intracellulare, M xenopi, M ulcerans*
- **Group IV – Rapid growers**
  - Capable of rapid growth, colonies developing within 7 days
  - E.g. *M fortuitum, M chelonae*

Ans: (c) M. avium

Ref: *Ananthanarayan, Paniker CJ, Textbook of Microbiology, 8th edition, London: John Wiley and Sons 2009, Page 360-61*

FORENSIC MEDICINE

1. A patient died due to jaundice. What will be the colour of corpse after embalming?

(a) Grey (b) Green

(c) Yellow (d) Brown

Explanation:

- Embalming of jaundiced corpses is problematic because **formalin** in embalming solutions react rapidly with **bilirubin** conjugates to give a mixture of uncharacterized **green pigments** that can impart a **Halloweenish hue** to the deceased.
- This can be avoided by using proprietary embalming solutions containing **glutaraldehyde** or **polymer-formaldehyde complexes**.

Color changes in skin and mucous membrane due to poisoning

- **Sulphuric and hydrochloric acid** – Gray, becoming black from blood
- **Nitric acid** – Brown or yellow
- **Hydrofluoric acid** – Reddish-brown
- **Carbolic acid** – Grayish-white
- **Oxalic acid –** Gray, blackened by blood*
- **Caustic alkalis** – Grayish-white
- **Mercuric chloride** – Bluish-white
- **Zinc chloride** – Whitish*
- **Chromic acid, potassium chromate** – Orange and leathery

Color of postmortem staining in some poisons

- **Carbon monoxide (CO)** – Cherry red*
- **Carbon dioxide (CO_2)** – Deep blue (reduced hemoglobin)*
- **Cyanide** – Bright red/pink*
- **Phosphorus or copper** – Dark brown/yellow
- **Hydrogen sulfide** – Bluish green*
- **Opiates** – Black
- **Nitrites, aniline, nitrobenzene, chlorates (methemoglobin formation)** – Chocolate or coffee-brown*

Ans: (c) Green

Ref: *McDonagh AF, Green Jaundice Revisited, Am J Med 2010 Sep;123(9):e23*

2. Calcium gluconate can be given in which acid poisoning?

(a) Sulphuric acid (b) Hydrofluoric acid

(c) Nitric acid (d) Carbolic acid

Explanation:

- **Calcium gluconate** is the antidote for poisons causing **hypocalcemia**
- Acids known to cause **hypocalcemia** are:

- **Oxalic acid**
- **Hydrofluoric acid**
- **Phosphoric acid**

Poisons causing hypocalcemia

- Oxalic acid
- Hydroflouric acid and Flourine
- Phosphoric acid and Phosphorus
- Ethylene glycol
- Cocaine
- Salicylates

Antidotes for common poisons

- **Acetaminophen** – N-acetyl cysteine*
- **Anticholinergics** (e.g., dhatura, atropine) – Physostigmine
- **Anticholinesterases** (e.g., OPCs) – Atropine and pralidoxime (2-PAM)
- **Benzodiazepines** – Flumazenil
- **Carbon monoxide** – Oxygen, hyperbaric oxygen
- **Cyanide** – Sodium nitrite, sodium thiosulfate*
- **Heavy metals** (lead, mercury, iron) and arsenic – Specific chelating agents
- **Methanol, ethylene glycol** – Ethanol or fomepizole
- **Opioids** – Naloxone

Ans: (b) Hydrofluoric acid

Ref: *VV Pillay, Modern Medical Toxicology, 4th edition, Page 44*

3. During cranial autopsy, facial incision is started at:

(a) At occiput
(b) Behind the ear lobe
(c) In front of the ear lobe
(d) At vertex

Explanation:

- For opening the skull, scalp is opened using a **coronal incision** which starts from the **mastoid process** just **behind one ear** and is carried over the vertex of the scalp to back of the opposite ear (**Intermastoidal incision).**

For opening the body cavities, there are **3 types of primary incisions:**

Incision	Extent	Preferred in
I shaped	Extends from chin straight down to symphysis pubis, passing either to left or right of umbilicus	**Most common**, in all cases
Y shaped	Bilateral incision beginning from a point close to acromial process and extends down below breast and across xiphoid process meeting in midline and extends to symphysis pubis similar to I shaped incision	In females, cosmetic reasons
Modified Y shaped	Incision begins from suprasternal notch to symphysis pubis similar to I shaped incision but is extended bilaterally from suprasternal notch over middle of clavicle over neck to behind the ear	Death due to pressure over neck (hanging, strangulation etc)

Ans: (b) Behind the ear lobe

Ref: *KSN Reddy, Essentials of Forensic Medicine, 33rd edition, Page 116*

4. While performing embalming, difficulty encountered due to arterial system problem. How should the embalming fluid be introduced to overcome this problem?

(a) Low pressure high velocity
(b) Low pressure low velocity
(c) High pressure high velocity
(d) High pressure low velocity

Explanation:

Embalming

- Injecting embalming fluid is to **delay putrefaction**
- Produces a permanent **chemical stiffening** similar to RM and normal rigor does not develop
- 70 kg body requires **10 litres**
- Best timing – **within 6 hours** of death
- Embalming should NOT be done before autopsy (disappearance of evidence – **201 IPC***)
    - Alters appearance of body, tissues and organs making it difficult to interpret any injury or disease
    - Completely destroys cyanide, alcohol
    - Blood grouping cannot be made out

Injection methods

(a) **Continuous Injection and Drainage**: Duration shortened but poor venous drainage and tissue saturation – Least Satisfactory*

(b) **Continuous Injection with Disrupted Drainage**

(c) **Alternate Injection and Drainage**

(d) **Discontinuous Injection and Drainage** – Repeated arterial injection at 2 hourly, venous drain tube which is kept closed – is opened a little before; kept open a little after starting another dose – Best Method*

Recommended fluid

- **Preservative**: Formalin, methanol
- **Germicide**: Phenol
- **Wetting agent**: Glycerin
- **Buffer**: Na Borate/Chlorate
- **Anticoagulant**: Sodium citrate
- **Dye**: Eosin
- **Perfume**: Oil of Wintergreen

Ans: (c) High pressure high velocity

Ref: *Ajmani ML, Embalming, Principles and Legal Aspects, 1st edition*

5. In hydrofluoric acid poisoning, which electrolyte abnormality is not seen?

(a) Hypernatremia
(b) Hypomagnesemia
(c) Hypocalcemia
(d) Hyperkalemia

Explanation:

Hydrofluoric acid poisoning

- Hydrofluoric acid is a unique acid, in that most of its toxicity is due to the **anion, fluoride**, and not to the cation, hydrogen.

MOA

- **Liquefactive necrosis*** (Unlike other inorganic acids)
- Decalcification and destruction of bone
- Production of insoluble salts of calcium and magnesium fluoride (resulting in hypocalcemia and hypomagnesemia)

Clinical features

- Local effect – Acid burns (1st to 3rd degree) with severe pain out of proportion to degree of burn (due to ability to traverse skin barrier and penetrate deeper tissue planes)
- **Systemic fluoride toxicity**
  - **Hypocalcaemia***
  - Hypomagnesaemia*
  - Hyperkalemia*
  - Metabolic acidosis*
  - Cardiac arrhythmias

Treatment

- First aid – Wash the area and immerse in iced solution of 25% magnesium sulfate
- Specific – **Calcium gluconate*** (locally and systemically) with **magnesium sulfate***

Ans: (a) Hypernatremia

Ref: *VV Pillay, Modern Medical Toxicology, 4th edition, Page 44*

6. Cephalic Index of 80-85 is seen in which of the following race?

(a) Mongols (b) Chinese

(c) European (d) Negroid

Explanation:

$$\text{Cephalic index} = \frac{\text{Maximum breadth of skull}}{\text{Maximum length of skull}} \times 100$$

- The length and breadth are measured by calipers between both parietal eminences, between glabella and external occipital protuberance, and not by measuring tape
- The skull of an Indian is Caucasian with a few Negroid characters
- With skull measurements, race can be determined in 85% = 90% of cases

Racial difference in the skull

Race	Type of Skull	Cephalic Index
Pure Aryans Aborigines Negroes	Dolichocephalic (long headed)	**70 – 75**
Europeans Chinese	Mesati-cephalic (Medium headed)	**75 – 80**
Mongolian	Brachy-cephalic (Short headed)	**80 – 85**

Ans: (a) Mongols

Ref: *The Essentials of Forensic Medicine and Toxicology by KS Narayan Reddy, 29th edition, 2010, Page 54*

7. Subpoena is a:

(a) Legal document
(b) Medicolegal document
(c) Medical document
(d) First information report (FIR)

Explanation:

SUBPOENA OR SUMMONS

- Section ***61 to 69 CrPC*** deals with summons.
- Subpoena means **Sub–Under**; **Poena – Penalty.**
- It is a **legal document** compelling the attendance of a witness in a Court of Law under penalty, or a particular day, time and place, for the purpose of giving evidence.
- It may also require him to bring with him any books, documents or other things under his control, that he is bound by law to produce as evidence.
- It is **issued by the Court in writing**, in duplicate, **signed** by the presiding officer of the Court and bears the seal of the Court.
- Crime number and name of the accused person is mentioned.
- It is served on the witness by a police officer, by a officer of the Court or other public servant by delivering one of the copies of summons.
- The person should sign a receipt on the back of the other copy.
- It can also be served by **registered post, or fixed on some conspicuous part of the house** in which the person resides.
- For **Government servants**, summons send in duplicate to the **head of the office** in which such person is employed.
- The witness will be excused from attending the Court, if he has a valid and urgent reason.
- **If witness fails to attend the court:**
  - In **Civil Case,** he or she is liable to pay damages.
  - In **Criminal Case**, he or she can be fined or court may issue bailable or non-bailable warrant.
- If witness is summoned by 2 courts one criminal and civil on the same day, he or she should attend criminal court and intimate the civil court of his inability to attend.
- If witness is summoned by 2 courts, higher court has priority over lower courts.
- If witness is summoned by 2 courts of same status, then priority is given for the summon he received first.

Ans: (a) Legal document

Ref: *The Essentials of Forensic Medicine and Toxicology by KS Narayan Reddy, 29th edition, 2010, Page 7*

PSM

1. A total of 130 patients were screened for disc prolapse by CT scan and confirmation of the disease was made by discectomy operation. Out of 56 patients who screened positive in CT scan, 46 were confirmed for disease in operation and the rest 74 patients who were screened negative in CT scan, only 40 patients were confirmed negative for the disease in operation. Calculate the positive and negative likelihood ratio:

(a) 2.875 and 0.531
(b) 6.07 and 1.12
(c) 1.12 and 6.07
(d) 0.531 and 2.875

Explanation:

The **likelihood Ratio (LR)** is the likelihood that a given test result would be expected in a patient with the target disorder compared to the likelihood that the same result would be expected in a patient without the target disorder.

$$\text{LR} = \frac{\textbf{Probability of finding in patients with disease}}{\textbf{Probability of same finding in patients without disease}}$$

- Likelihood ratios (LR) in medical testing are used to interpret diagnostic tests.
- Basically, the LR tells us **how likely a patient has a disease or condition**.
- The higher the ratio, the **more likely** they have the **disease or condition**.
- Tests can be either positive or negative, so there are two ratios:

Positive LR:

$$\textbf{Positive LR} = \frac{\textbf{Probability of person with the condition tests positive}}{\textbf{Probability a person without the condition tests positive}}$$

Negative LR:

$$\textbf{Negative LR} = \frac{\textbf{Probability of person with the condition tests negative}}{\textbf{Probability a person without the condition tests negative}}$$

- Sensitivity and specificity are an alternative way to define the likelihood ratio:
    - **Positive LR = sensitivity / (100 – specificity).**
    - **Negative LR = (100 – sensitivity) / specificity.**

Screening test (CT Scan) results	Diagnostic test (**Discectomy operation)**		**Total**
	Diseased	**Not diseased**	
Positive	46 (True positive)	10 (False positive)	56
Negative	34 (False Negative)	40 (True negative)	74
	80	50	130

Sensitivity = TP/ TP+FN = 46/46+34 = 46/80 = 0.575

Specificity = TN/ TN+FP = 40/40+10 = 40/50 = 0.8

Positive LR = Sensitivity / (100 – specificity) = 2.875

Negative LR = (100 – sensitivity) / specificity = 0.531

$$\text{Positive LR} = \frac{\text{Probability of person with the condition tests positive}}{\text{Probability a person without the condition tests positive}}$$

$$= \frac{46/80}{10/50}$$

$$= 2.875$$

$$\text{Negative LR} = \frac{\text{Probability of person with the condition tests negative}}{\text{Probability a person without the condition tests negative}}$$

$$= \frac{34/80}{40/50}$$

$$= 0.531$$

Ans: (a) 2.875 and 0.531

Ref: *Fundamentals of Evidence-Based Medicine, Author: Kameshwar Prasad, 2nd edition 2013, Page 100*

2. Which of the following option is true about ROC curve:

(a) It is a method of evaluating the quality or performance of screening tests

(b) It is plotted as test sensitivity as x coordinate versus its 1- specificity or false positive rate (FPR) as the y coordinate

(c) A perfect test has an area under the ROC curve (AUROCC) of 1

(d) A decrease in sensitivity results in decrease in specificity

Explanation:

Receiver Operating Characteristic (ROC) Curve

- The receiver operating characteristic (ROC) curve, is defined as a **plot of test sensitivity as the y coordinate versus its 1-specificity or false positive rate (FPR) as the x coordinate**.
- It is an effective method of evaluating the **quality or performance of diagnostic tests**.
- Evaluation of diagnostic tests is a matter of concern in modern medicine not only for confirming the presence of disease but also to rule out the disease in healthy subjects.
- In practice, we choose a cutoff level above which we consider the test to be **Positive** and below which we consider the test to be **Negative**.
- ROC curve helps us to decide this cutoff level.
- Receiver Operating Characteristic (ROC) curves plot the sensitivity of a test versus its false positive rate (1-Specificity) for various Cut-off points.
- A decrease in sensitivity results in increase in specificity.
- An ROC curve is based on the notion of a "separator" scale, the complete separation of the two underlying distributions implies a perfectly discriminating test while complete overlap implies no discrimination.
- The plot of True Positive Factor (TPF) (sensitivity) versus False Positive Factor (FPF)/(1-specificity) across varying cut-offs generates a curve in the unit square called an ROC curve.
- **Test accuracy:** The closer the graph is to the top and left-hand borders, the more accurate the test. Likewise, the closer the graph to the diagonal, the less accurate the test. A perfect test would go straight from zero upto the top-left corner and then straight across the horizontal.

- **Test accuracy** is also shown as the **area under the curve**. The greater the area under the curve, the more accurate the test. A perfect test has an area under the ROC curve (AUROCC) of 1. The diagonal line in a ROC curve represents perfect chance. The area under the diagonal is .5 (half of the area of the graph).

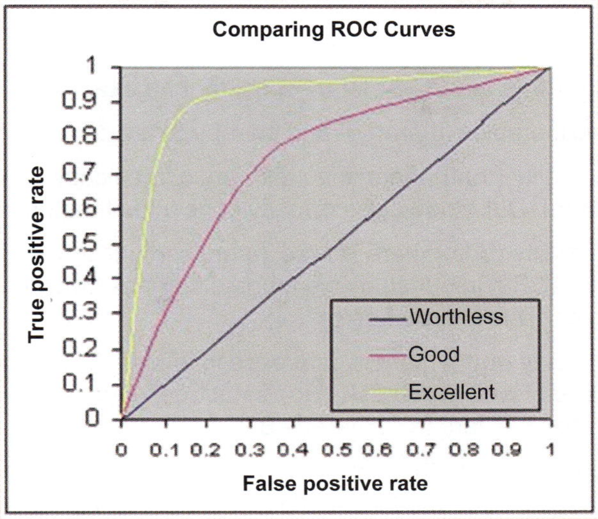

Ans: (c) A perfect test has an area under the ROC curve (AUROCC) of 1

Ref: *Chapman and Hall/CRC Biostatistics Series, Statistical Evaluation of Diagnostic Performance: Topics in ROC Analysis, 2012, Page 6*

3. What happens to sample size when range of allowable error is doubled?

(a) Reduced to 1/4
(b) Reduced to 1/2
(c) Sample size does not depend on acceptable error
(d) Cannot to be calculated

Explanation:

- Calculation of exact sample size is an important part of research design.
- When the **sample size (n)** is very **small**, statistical significance is **not** achieved even though clinical significance exists (**type II error, i.e., accept Null hypothesis** Ho when alternate hypothesis H1 is true).
- When sample size (n) is too big, strong statistical significance is achieved even though that difference was not clinically meaningful (type I error, i.e., reject Null hypothesis Ho when Ho is true).
- Thus, there is a need of calculation of sample size for conducting any study.
- For **quantitative data,** the formula for sample size **$n = 4\ SD^2 / E^2$.**

Where,

SD = **Standard deviation** in a population known from past experience/study.

E = **Allowable error** which may be absolute or relative.

Example: Mean pulse rate of a population is believed to be 70/minutes with standard deviation of 8 beats. Calculate the minimum size of the sample to verify this, if allowable error = ± 1 beat at 5% risk.

$n = 4\ SD^2 / E^2$

n = $4 \times 8 \times 8 / 1 \times 1 = 256$

If E = **± 2 beats with 5% risk**

n = $4 \times 8 \times 8 / 2 \times 2 = 64$

Ans: (a) Reduced to 1/4

Ref: *Methods in Biostatistics by BK Mahajan, 9th edition, Page 124*

4. Rejection of true Null Hypothesis:

(a) Type II error
(b) Type I error
(c) Both
(d) None

Explanation:

To understand types of error in any study, let us consider one example:

Two groups receiving two therapies (therapy A and therapy B) are compared. 4 possible outcomes are possible:

- It is possible that in reality (truth) there is no difference in efficacy between therapy A and therapy B [Null hypothesis (Ho) is true]. Our study also correctly concludes that the two groups do not differ.
- It is possible that in reality (truth) there is no difference in efficacy between therapy A and therapy B [Null hypothesis (Ho) is true]. But in our study we found difference between the groups, i.e., there is difference between the therapies. This is **type I error*.**
- It is possible that in reality (truth) there is difference in efficacy between therapy A and therapy B [Alternate hypothesis (H1) is true or Null hypothesis (Ho) is not true]. Our study also correctly concludes that the two groups differ or therapy A differs from therapy B.
- It is possible that in reality (truth) there is difference in efficacy between therapy A and therapy B [Alternate hypothesis (H1) is true or Null hypothesis (Ho) is not true]. But in our study we found that there is no difference between therapy A and therapy B. This is **type II error***.

		REALITY	
		Treatments are NOT different	**Treatments are different**
Possible Conclusions	**We conclude treatments are NOT different from each other**	Correct decision (cell a)	**Type II error** (probability = β) (cell b)
	We conclude treatments are different from each other	**Type I error** (probability = α) (cell c)	Correct decision (cell d)

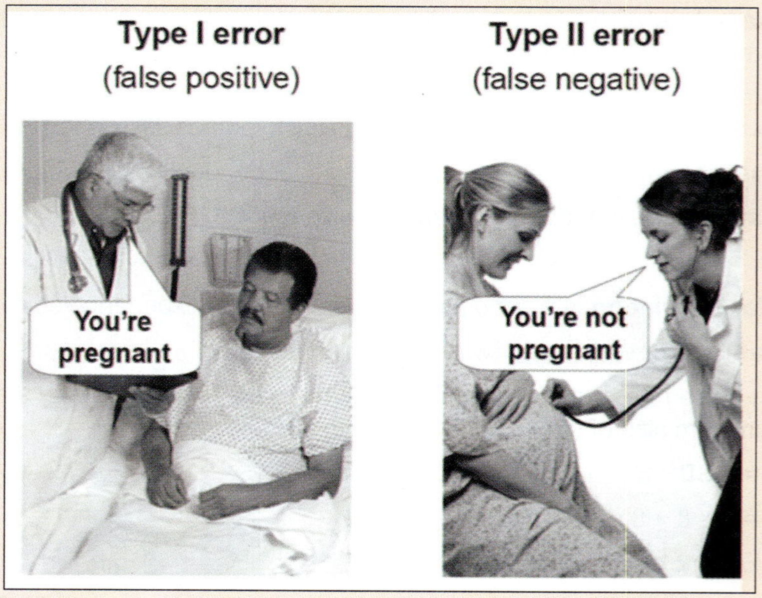
Type I error
(false positive)
Type II error
(false negative)
You're pregnant
You're not pregnant

Ans: (b) Type I error

Ref: *Gordis Epidemiology, 6th edition, Page 218*

5. Allowed amount of chlorine in drinking water:

(a) 2 ppm (b) 0.5 ppm

(c) 1.5 ppm (d) 4 ppm

Explanation:

Chlorination

- Water is disinfected by oxidizing chemical like chlorine and its compound to make it fit for drinking purpose.
- **Chlorination:** When chlorine is added to water, it forms hydrochloric acid and hypochlorous acid. Hypochlorous acid further dissociates into hydrogen ions (H^+) and hypochlorite ions (OCl^-).

  $Cl + H_2O = HCl + HOCl$ $HOCl = H^+ + OCl^-$
- The reaction is reversible. The disinfection action of chlorine is mainly by hypochlorous acid and partly due to hypochlorite ion.

Chlorine Demand:

- The difference between the **amount of chlorine added to water** and the **amount of residual chlorine** after a specified contact period (**usually 60 minutes**), at a given temperature and PH of water, is defined as **"chlorine demand".**
- When chlorine is added to water, it attacks organic matter and attempt to destroy organism.
- If enough chlorine is added, some will remain in the water after all possible organisms have been destroyed. What is left is called free chlorine.
- Free chlorine will remain in the water and is used to destroy new contamination.
- So, if water is tested and found to contain some free chlorine, it proves that the most dangerous organisms in the water have been removed and it is likely to be safe to drink. This process is called measuring the chlorine residual.
- For normal domestic use, residual chlorine levels at the point where the consumer collects water should be between **0.2 and 0.5 mg/l.** The higher level will be close to the disinfection point.

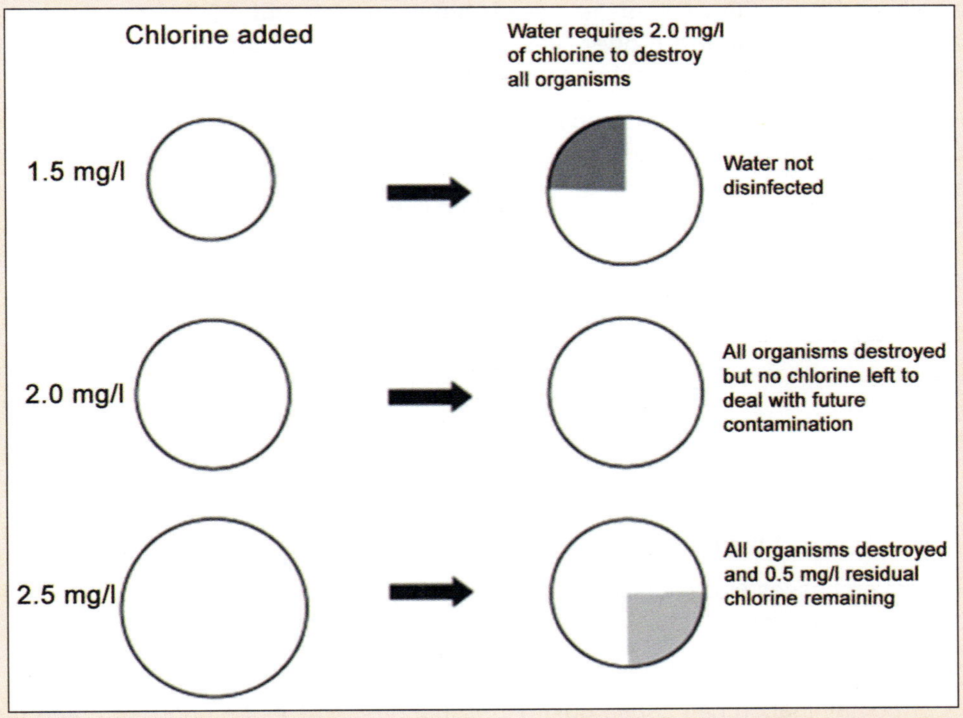

Figure: The effect of chlorine residual

Superchlorination:

- When there is potential danger of outbreak of intestinal infections or when water is heavily polluted or fluctuates rapidly in quality, large doses of chlorine is added to water and it is called superchlorination. Here, free residual chlorine is **1-2 ppm**, after breakpoint.

Dechlorination:

- Excess of free available chlorine is removed before water is consumed by adding two tablets (each **0.5 gm)** of sodium thiosulfate per **500 liters** of water. It is done usually after superchlorination.
- A contact for a minimum **15 minutes** should be allowed.

Ans: (b) 0.5 ppm

Ref: *WHO (2004) Guidelines for Drinking Water Quality, 3rd edition., WHO, Geneva, Page 107, CDC Guidelines*

6. What is saturation index?

(a) It is used to assess the quality of air by measuring concentration of pollutants

(b) It is used to assess the quality of water by estimating hardness, total dissolved solids, alkalinity and PH

(c) It is used to assess the quality of soil that whether it is good for growing crops

(d) It is used to assess the quality of milk by estimating the bacterial count in it

Explanation:

SATURATION INDEX

- The Saturation Index (SI) is a method of determining whether **water will deposit calcium carbonate** or **maintain it in solution**. In short it tells us whether water is **corrosive or scale forming.**
- The **SI incorporates the five balance factors:** pH, total alkalinity, calcium hardness, temperature, and total dissolved solids.
- For balanced water the value of the index is **between - 0.3 and + 0.3**. Corrosive water is - 0.4 and lower. Scaling water is **+ 0.4 and higher**. Values close to **zero** indicate that the water is balanced and there should not be problems from either corrosion or scaling.
- Having water outside of the balanced range can contribute to **extensive damage** to the pool surface, equipment and structure.

Saturation Index (SI) Table		
Saturation Index (SI)	**Description**	**Recommendations**
-3.0 – 5.0	Very Severe Corrosion	Treatment Recommended
-1.0 to -3.0	Moderate Corrosion	Consider Treatment
0.0	Balanced	Treatment Not Needed
1.0 to 3.0	Moderate Scale	Consider Treatment
3.0 to 5.0	Very Severe Scale	Treatment Recommended

CORROSION

- Corrosion is one of the most common problems affecting domestic water supplies.
- Chemical processes slowly dissolve metal, causing plumbing pipes, fixtures and water-using equipment to deteriorate and fail.
- Copper or other metals oxidize in a process and can leach into tap water.
- Copper contamination can cause gastrointestinal problems in the short term and damage the liver and kidneys over time.

- Lead contamination can cause physical and mental development problems in children. In adults, it can lead to high blood pressure and kidney problems.
- The rate of corrosion depends on many factors including the water's pH, electrical conductivity, oxygen concentration and temperature.
- **pH of water:** Soft water that contains sodium salts does not coat the pipes and consequently is more corrosive. Water that is moderately alkaline (40 to 70 mg/L) with a pH between 7.0 and 8.2 is usually not corrosive. Water with a pH below 6.5 will be corrosive, especially if alkalinity also is low.
- **Alkalinity of Water:** Total alkalinity refers to the total bases in water that can neutralize acid. These include bicarbonates, carbonates, hydroxides, and some phosphates and silicates. Alkalinity is reported in milligrams per liter of calcium carbonate.

  Water that contains calcium or magnesium salts (hard water) is less corrosive, because the minerals that cause hard water tend to coat and protect the inside of pipes.
- **High Dissolved Solids and Electrical Conductivity:** Minerals dissolved in water separate into charged particles (ions) that conduct electricity. Conductivity is a problem only when water has a high mineral content; pure water does not conduct electricity. Galvanic corrosion occurs at or very near the joint between the two metals. Every joint where different metals connect is a potential site for galvanic corrosion if the water has high amounts of dissolved minerals.
- **Dissolved Oxygen and Other Gases:** Oxygen dissolved in water is a primary corrosive agent. Water exposed to the air absorbs oxygen. Oxygen in rain and surface water is usually removed when water seeps into the ground; deep wells are usually oxygen free. In contrast, shallow wells and surface water often contain more oxygen.
- **Water Temperature:** Corrosion is more likely and more rapid at higher water temperatures. The rate of corrosion triples or quadruples as water temperature rises from 60°F to 140°F. Above 140°F, the rate of corrosion doubles for every 20°F increase.

Treating the water can reduce corrosion to acceptable levels, but generally will not eliminate it. Treatment method depends on what causes the corrosion.

For treating the acidity: Chips of calcium carbonate (limestone), marble, magnesia (magnesium carbonate), or other alkaline materials should be dissolved to neutralize the water.

Acid-neutralizing filters are usually installed after the pressure tank. As water flows through the filter, pH increases which decreases corrosivity.

For Reducing salts: Removing high concentrations of dissolved salts from water requires a reverse osmosis system. Reverse osmosis can remove 80 to 95 percent of salts from the water entering the system.

For Reducing dissolved oxygen: Installing a flexible membrane or a floating disc in the pressure tank will minimize the water's contact with air.

Ans: (b) It is used to assess the quality of water by estimating hardness, total dissolved solids, alkalinity and PH

Ref: *Oram, B. Corrosion, Saturation Index, Balanced Water in Drinking Water Systems, 2009, Wilkes University Center for Environmental Quality, Wilkes-Barre, PA*

7. After 10 days of antibiotics patient came back again with complaints of diarrhea. Which of the following statement is true?

(a) Hand scrub with alcohol based antiseptics is superior to hand washing with soap and water

(b) Hand washing should be done only with clean water

(c) Hand washing with hot water is superior than cold water

(d) Antiseptic detergents are better than alcohol based hand rubs

Explanation:

"Hand scrub with alcohol based antiseptics is superior to hand washing with soap and water." – **Ref:** *WHO Guidelines on Hand Hygiene in Health Care and Am J Trop Med Hyg. 2010 Feb; 82(2): 270-278*

INDICATIONS OF HAND WASHING

a. Wash hands with soap and water when visibly dirty or visibly soiled with blood or other body fluids or after using the toilet.

b. If exposure to potential spore-forming pathogens is strongly suspected or proven, including outbreaks of C. difficile, hand washing with soap and water is the preferred means.

c. Use an alcohol-based handrub as the preferred means for routine hand antisepsis, if hands are not visibly soiled.

d. If alcohol-based handrub is not obtainable, wash hands with soap and water.

e. Perform hand hygiene:

- Before and after touching the patient.
- Before handling an invasive device for patient care, regardless of whether or not gloves are used.
- After contact with body fluids or excretions, mucous membranes, non-intact skin, or wound dressings.
- If moving from a contaminated body site to another body site during care of the same patient after contact with inanimate surfaces and objects (including medical equipment) in the immediate vicinity of the patient.
- After removing sterile or non-sterile gloves.

f. Before handling medication or preparing food perform hand hygiene using an alcohol-based handrub or wash hands with antimicrobial soap and water.

HAND HYGIENE TECHNIQUE

a. Apply a palmful of alcohol-based handrub and cover all surfaces of the hands. Rub hands until dry. Duration of the entire procedure: 20-30 seconds.

b. When washing hands with soap and water, wet hands with water and apply the amount of product necessary to cover all surfaces. Rinse hands with water and dry thoroughly with a single-use towel. Use clean, running water whenever possible. Duration of the entire procedure: 40-60 seconds.

c. Avoid using hot water, as repeated exposure to hot water may increase the risk of dermatitis.

d. Use a towel to turn off tap/faucet. Dry hands thoroughly using a method that does not recontaminate hands. Make sure towels are not used multiple times or by multiple people.

e. Liquid, bar, leaf or powdered forms of soap are acceptable. When bar soap is used, small bars of soap in racks that facilitate drainage should be used to allow the bars to dry.

(See Figures on the next pages)

Ans: (a) Hand scrub with alcohol based antiseptics is superior to hand washing with soap and water

Ref: *WHO Guidelines on Hand Hygiene in Health Care: A Summary. First Global Patient Safety Challenge Clean Care is Safer Care. World Health Organization 2009 and Am J Trop Med Hyg 2010 Feb; 82(2): 270-278*

Hand Hygiene Technique with Alcohol-Based Formulation

Duration of the entire procedure: 20-30 seconds

1a

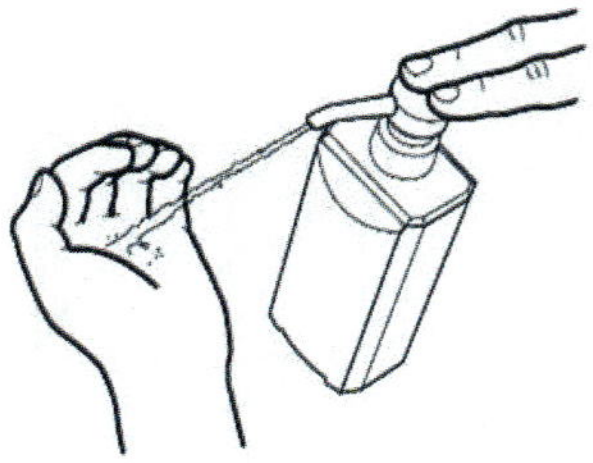

1b

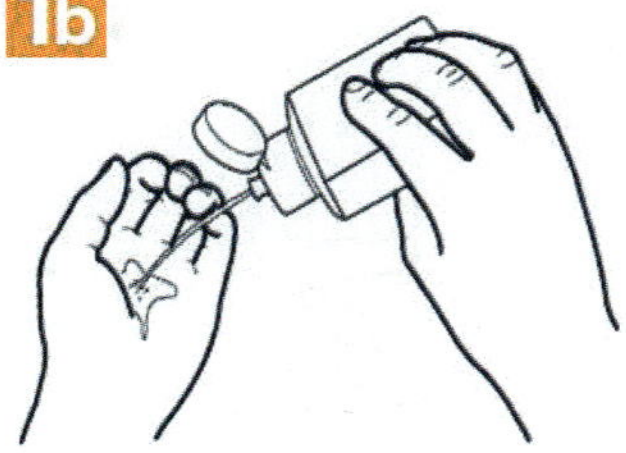

Apply a palmful of the product in a cupped hand, covering all surfaces

2

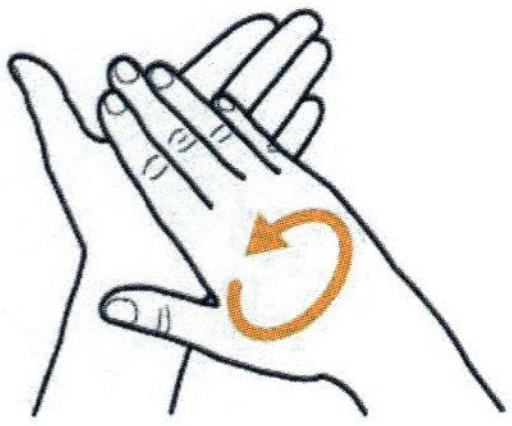

Rub hands palm to palm

3

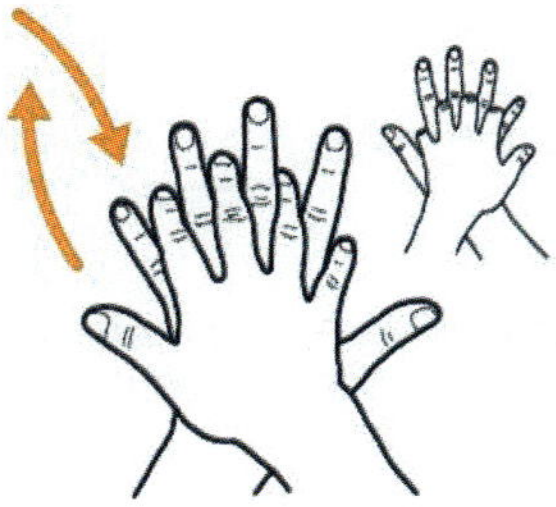

Right palm over left dorsum with interlaced fingers and vice versa

4

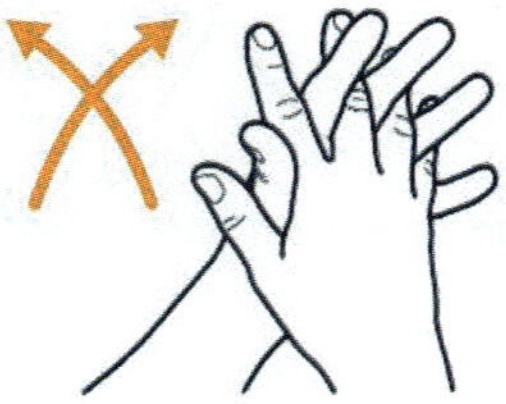

Palm to palm with fingers interlaced

5

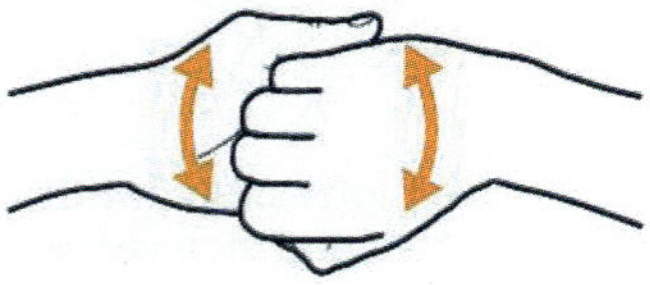

Backs of fingers to opposing palms with fingers interlocked

6

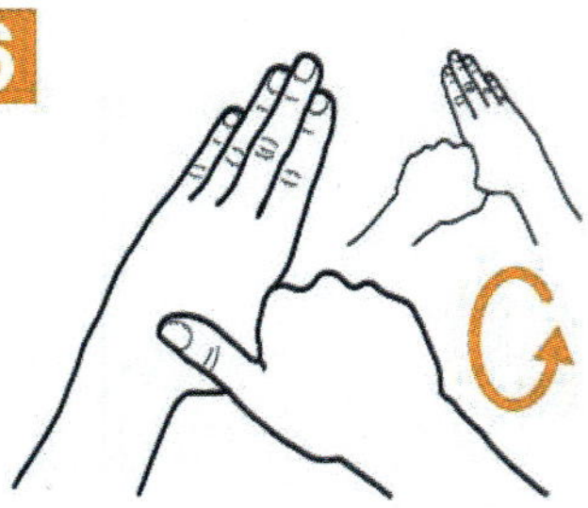

Rotational rubbing of left thumb clasped in right palm and vice versa

7

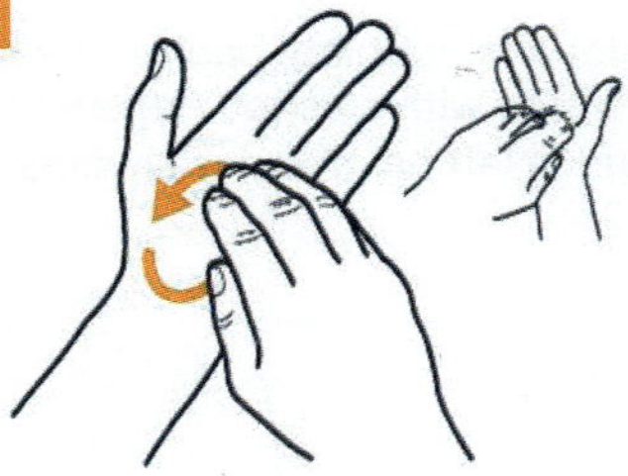

Rotational rubbing, backwards and forwards with clasped fingers of right hand in left palm and vice versa

8

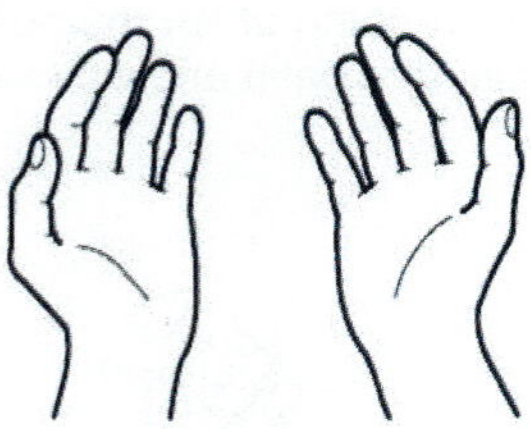

Once dry, your hands are safe

Hand Hygiene Technique with Soap and Water

Duration of the entire procedure: 40-60 seconds

0

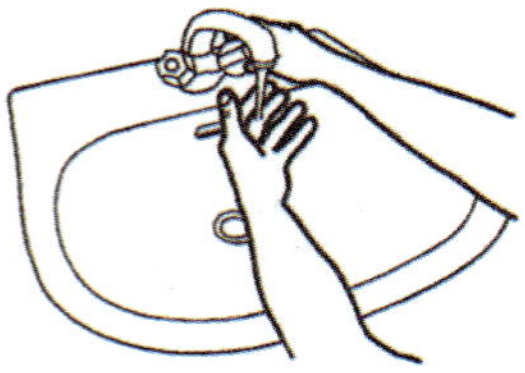

Wet hands with water

1

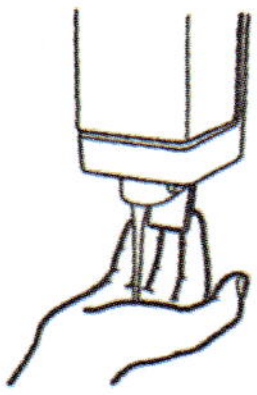

Apply enough soap to cover all hand surfaces

2

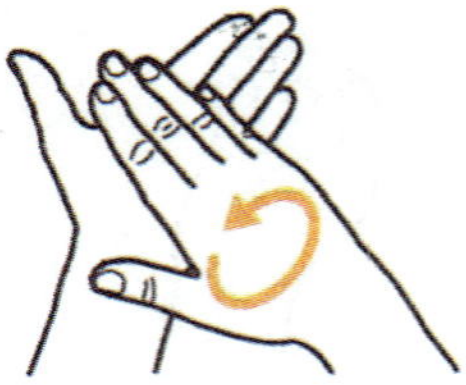

Rub hands palm to palm

3

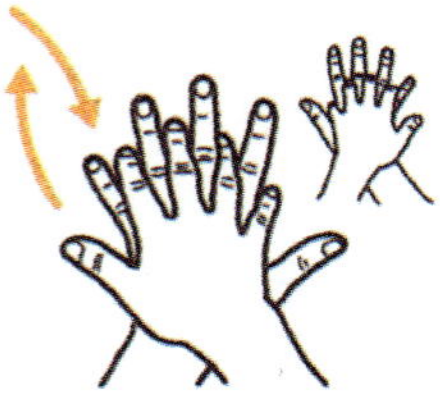

Right palm over left dorsum with interlaced fingers and vice versa

4

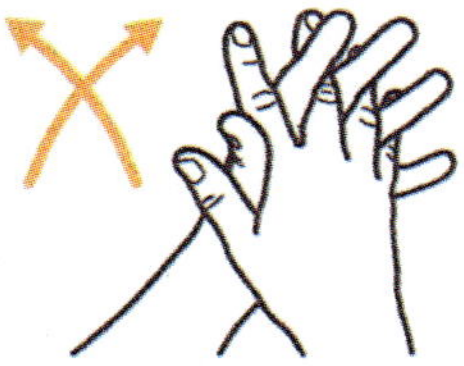

Palm to palm with fingers interlaced

5

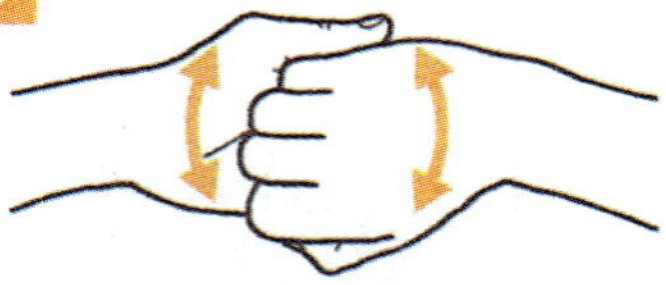

Backs of fingers to opposing palms with fingers interlocked

6

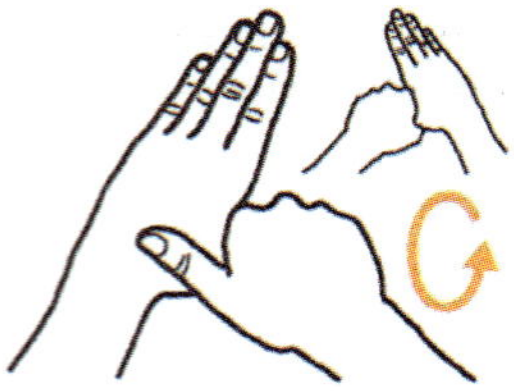

Rotational rubbing of left thumb clasped in right palm and vice versa

7

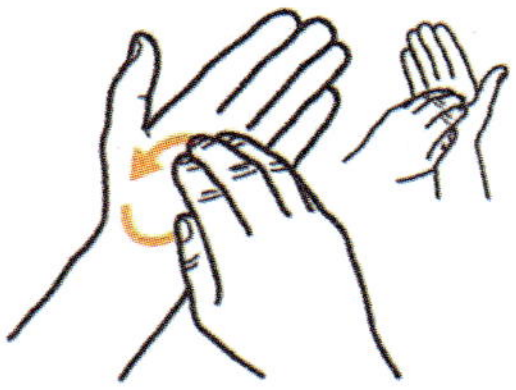

Rotational rubbing, backwards and forwards with clasped fingers of right hand in left palm and vice versa

8

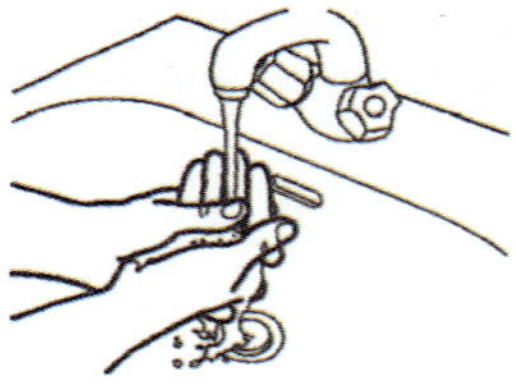

Rinse hands with water

9

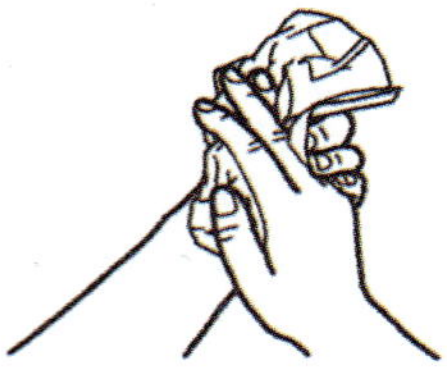

Dry hands thoroughly with a single use towel

10

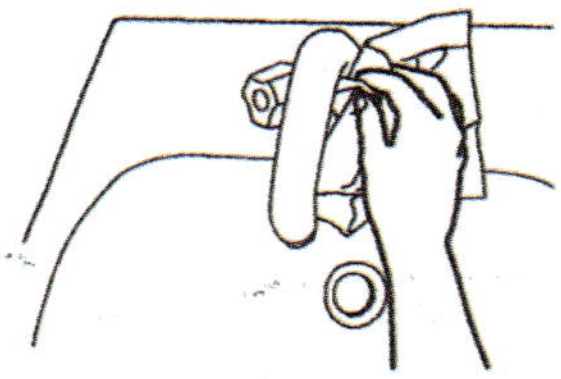

Use towel to turn off faucet

11

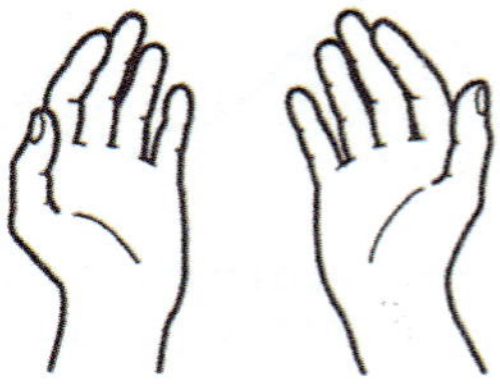

Your hands are now safe

8. Median incubation period means:

(a) Time for 50% cases to occur

(b) Time between primary case and secondary case

(c) Time between onset of infection and period of maximum infectivity

(d) Median of several incubation period

Explanation:

Median Incubation Period

- It is relevant in **common source single exposure epidemic/point source epidemic**.
- This is an important part of understanding natural history of the disease.
- This implies **average incubation period**.

Serial Interval

- The gap in time between the onset of the primary case and the secondary case is called the "**serial interval**". This helps to measure incubation period.

Generation Time

- Time between onset of infection and period of maximum infectivity is "**generation time**".
- It is roughly equivalent to **incubation period**.
- It refers to transmissions of infection, whether clinical or subclinical. However, incubation period is used only for manifest disease.

ALSO NOTE:

Incubation period	Between invasion by an infectious agent and appearance of the first sign / symptoms
Median incubation period	The time required for 50 percent of the cases to occur following exposure
Latent period	Equal to IP in non-communicable disease
Serial interval	Between onset of primary case and secondary case
Generation time	Interval between the receipt of infection by a host and maximal infectivity
Period of communicability	During which an infectious agent can be communicated

Ans: (a) Time for 50% cases to occur

Ref: *Textbook of Preventive and Social Medicine, K Park, 22nd edition, Page 62*

9. Human developmental index includes all except:

(a) Adult literacy

(b) Per capita income

(c) Life expectancy

(d) Infant mortality rate

Explanation:

Composite index of quality of life	
Physical Quality of Life Index (PQLI)	Consolidates three indicators: • **Infant mortality** • **Life expectancy at age one** • **Literacy** Range – **0 to 100**

Contd.

Contd.

Human Developmental Index (HDI)	Consolidates three indicators: • **Life expectancy at birth (Longevity)** • **Adult literacy rate and mean year of schooling (Knowledge)** • **Real GDP per capita (Income)** **Notes:** ○ Extra indicator as compared to PQLI is income ○ Infant mortality and life expectancy at age one is conceptually clubbed in HDI as life expectancy at birth Range – **0 to 1**

Ans: (d) Infant mortality rate

Ref: *Park 'Textbook of Preventive and Social Medicine', 22nd edition, Page 16*

10. In a prospective study, 1200 patients were randomly selected to study the effect of a new drug. The drug will be given for 5 years and its association with cataract will be studied. What type of study is this?

(a) Case control study
(b) Cohort study
(c) Randomized clinical trial
(d) Cross sectional study

Explanation:

COHORT STUDY

- A type of analytical study used for **hypothesis testing**
- Proceeds from **cause to effect**
- Starts with risk factor or suspected cause
- Involves **longer number** subjects
- **Long follow up** period needed
- Identifies **several diseases due to a single risk factor**
- Yields **incidence rate, relative risk, attributable risk**
- Expensive
- **Less chance of bias**

Smoking	Developed lung cancer	Did not develop lung cancer	Total
Yes	a	b	a+b
No	c	d	c+d

- Incidence rate among smokers = a/(a+b)
- Incidence rate among non-smokers = c/(c+d)

$$\text{Relative risk} = \frac{\text{Incidence of disease among exposed}}{\text{Incidence of disease among non-exposed}}$$

RELATIVE RISK

- Relative risk is the **ratio** of incidence of disease among exposed and the incidence among non-exposed
- Estimation of relative risk is important in **etiological enquiries**
- It is a direct **measure of strength of the association between** the suspected cause and effect
- **Relative risk of 1 indicates no association**
- Greater than **one** indicates **positive association**

ATTRIBUTABLE RISK (RISK DIFFERENCE)

- Difference in the **incidence rate** between an **exposed group** and a **non-exposed group**
- Suggests the amount of the disease that might be eliminated if the factor under study could be eliminated

$$\frac{\text{Incidence of disease among exposed} - \text{Incidence of disease among non-exposed}}{\text{Incidence rate among exposed}} \times 100$$

POPULATION ATTRIBUTABLE RISK

- Incidence of disease in the **total population** minus among those who were **not exposed**
- Estimate of the amount that the disease could be reduced in the population if the suspected factor is controlled

Advantages of Cohort Study

- **Incidence** can be calculated
- **Several possible outcomes** related to exposure can be studied simultaneously
- **Relative risk** can be estimated
- **Dose-response ratios** can be calculated

Disadvantages of Cohort Study

- Involves **large number** of people
- Unsuitable for investigating **uncommon diseases** or diseases with **low incidence**
- It takes a **long time** to complete the study and obtain results
- Difficult to keep a large number of individuals under medical surveillance indefinitely
- **Administrative problems** – Loss of experienced staff, loss of funding, extensive record keeping is inevitable
- A substantial proportion of original cohort **can be lost** – they may migrate, lose interest
- Selection of comparison groups which are representative of the exposed and unexposed groups
- There may be changes in the standard methods or diagnostic criteria of disease over prolonged follow-up
- **Expensive**
- The study itself may after behavior of the cohort
- Ethical problems

Examples

- **Prospective cohort studies:** Framingham Heart study, Study of OCPs and Health by Royal College of General Practitioners, Doll and Hills Study on Smoking and Lung Cancer
- **Retrospective cohort studies:** Roles of Arsenic in human carcinogenesis, mortality of groups of physicians in relation to exposure to radiation, polyvinyl chloride in liver angiosarcoma

Ans: (b) Cohort study

Ref: *Park's Textbook of Preventive and Social Medicine, 23rd edition*

ENT

1. Identify the marked structure in the below picture:

(a) Ampulla

(b) Saccule

(c) Endolymphatic sac

(d) Utricle

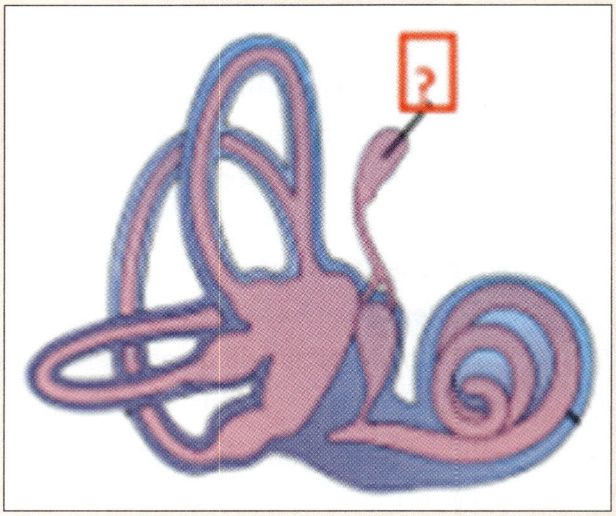

Explanation:

- The marked part is the **endolymphatic sac**
- The **endolymph** gets absorbed **here**
- The sac is the **dilated terminal portion** of the **endolymphatic duct** and lies between the two layers of **dura** on the posterior surface of the **petrous bone**
- The sac is **dilated** in **Meniere's disease***
- The surgical treatment of Meniere's disease involves **decompression or drainage of this sac**
- The **surgical landmark** for endolymphatic sac is the **'Donaldson's line'**, which is an imaginary like running parallel to the horizontal semicircular canal bisecting the posterior semicircular canal. The sac lays Inferior to this line

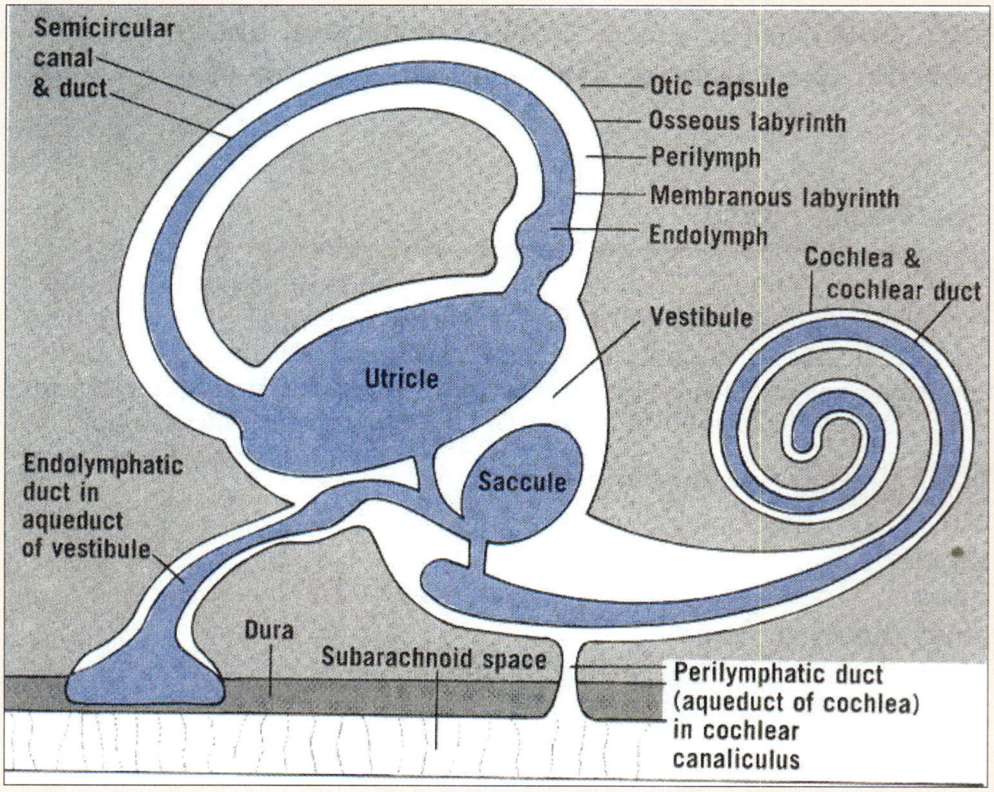

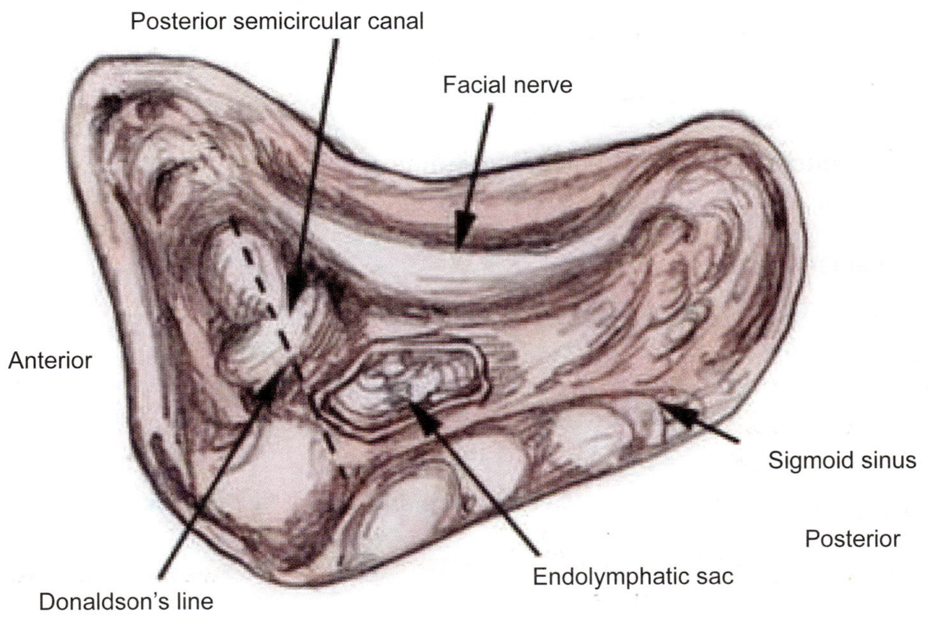

Ans: (c) Endolymphatic sac

Ref: *Diseases of the Ear, Nose and Throat by PL Dhingra, 6th edition, 2014, Page 9*

2. Which of the following is a contraindication for cochlear implant?

(a) Mondini dysplasia
(b) Michael aplasia
(c) Scheibe dysplasia
(d) Alexander dysplasia

Explanation:

Michael Aplasia

- Characterized by **Total absence of both the bony and membranous labyrinth*.**
- Hence no hearing aid or cochlear implant is feasible in these patients.
- The outer and middle ear may however be normal in these patients.

Bing-Siebenmann Dysplasia

- Characterized by complete absence of **membranous labyrinth*.**
- So, cochlear implant is not feasible.

Mondini Dysplasia

- Only **basal coil of the cochlea** is present.
- It can be unilateral or bilateral.
- May be seen in association with:
  - **Pendred syndrome**
  - **Treacher-Collins syndrome**
  - **Waardenburg syndrome**

Scheibe Dysplasia

- Also called **cochleosaccular dysplasia.**
- Only **cochlea and saccule** are affected.
- It is the **most common inner ear abnormality***
- Inherited as **autosomal recessive non-syndromic** trait.
- The bony labyrinth, Utricle and semicircular canals are **normal.**

Alexander Dysplasia

- Only the basal turn of the cochlea is affected.
- This part of the cochlea is for **high frequency hearing**, therefore the patient has only **high frequency deafness** and residual hearing in low frequencies is maintained.

Ans: (b) Michael aplasia

Ref: *Diseases of the Ear, Nose and Throat by PL Dhingra, 6th edition, 2014, Page 115*

3. Oroantral fistula is caused by all the following except:

(a) Dental extraction (b) Carcinoma of maxilla
(c) Caldwell Luc operation (d) Maxillectomy

Explanation:

Oroantral fistula

- Oroantral fistula is a communication between the **maxillary antrum and oral cavity.**
- In **maxillectomy** the maxilla is removed and therefore there is no possibility of forming an oroantral fistula.
- The opening is generally situated on the **alveolus** or the **gingivolabial sulcus.**
- **Causes of Oroantral fistula:**
  - **Dental extraction – Most common*** especially upper **first premolar and molars** as their roots are closely related to the maxillary antrum
  - Erosion due to **malignancy**
  - Trauma due to **penetrating injuries**
  - **Osteitis** of maxilla
  - Failure of sub-labial incision to heal after **Caldwell-Luc surgery**
- The treatment includes repair by **buccal or palatal flap**. The disease in the maxillary sinus is cleared via **Caldwell-Luc surgery**.
- Please note–Caldwell-Luc surgery is used for repairing an **oroantral fistula**; however an improperly done Caldwell-Luc surgery can also cause it.

Ans: (d) Maxillectomy

Ref: *Diseases of the Ear, Nose and Throat by PL Dhingra, 6th edition, 2014, Page 186*

4. Ethmoid polyp is characterized by all the following, except:

(a) Viral in origin (b) Multiple
(c) Antihistamines usefulr (d) Surgery is treatment of choice

Explanation:

Ethmoidal Nasal Polyps

- **Nasal polyps** are non-neoplastic masses of edematous mucosa.
- The etiology is linked to:
  - Inflammatory conditions of the nose (**Rhinosinusitis**)
  - Disorders of ciliary motility (**Kartagener and Young syndrome**)
  - Thick mucus secretions (**Cystic fibrosis**)
- **Samter's triad** consists of:
  - **Nasal polyps**
  - **Asthma**
  - **Aspirin intolerance**
- Since these polyps arise from the **ethmoidal sinus**, which are **multiple**, the polyps are also multiple.
- **Antihistaminics** will only help in reducing the allergic symptoms, which are generally associated with ethmoidal polyps.
- **Intranasal steroid sprays** are useful in reducing the symptoms and also help in reducing the recurrence rate.
- **Surgical treatment** gives instant relief and is indicated in extensive polyps and in patients who are not willing or have a contraindication to medical therapy with steroids.

Ans: (a) Viral in origin

Ref: *Diseases of the Ear, Nose and Throat by PL Dhingra, 6th edition, 2014,* Page 172

5. Which among the following is not true about otosclerosis?

(a) Hearing better in louder conditions
(b) Eustachian tube is always abnormal
(c) Tympanic membrane is normal
(d) Bilateral progressive conductive deafness

Explanation:

- **Eustachian tube function** is **normal** in **otosclerosis***

OTOSCLEROSIS

- **Irregular spongy bone** replaces the **dense endochondral layer** of the **bony labyrinth**
- Hereditary
- Associated with ***Van der Hoove's* syndrome**
  - **Osteogenesis imperfecta**
  - **Otosclerosis** and
  - **Blue sclera**
- More common in **females**
- Hearing loss **worsens** during **pregnancy**
- **Cochlear type** presents with **SNHL**
- **Stapedial type** has COHL and may have anterior (most common) posterior, circumferential, biscuit or obliterative focus
- **Symptoms**: **Hearing loss**, **Paracusis willisi** and **tinnitus** (indicates an active focus)

- **Signs: Schwartze sign***– Reddish hue over the promontory because of increased vasculature in active lesions
- PTA will show the type of hearing loss and **Carhart's** notch which is a dip in the bone conduction at 2kHz
- Impedance audiometry will show a **'As' type curve**
- Medical treatment with **sodium fluoride** can be tried
- **Surgery** is the **treatment of choice** and includes **stapedotomy or stapedectomy** followed by replacement with a piston made of Teflon or stainless steel or titanium

Ans: (b) Eustachian tube is always abnormal

Ref: *Diseases of the Ear, Nose and Throat by PL Dhingra, 5th edition, 2010, Page 98*

6. Posterior ethmoidal sinus drains into:

(a) Sphenoethmoidal recess (b) Superior meatus
(c) Inferior meatus (d) Middle meatus

Explanation:

Lateral Wall of Nose

- Lateral wall of nose – has **3 turbinates – superior, middle and inferior**.
  - **Inferior** turbinate is a **separate bone**.
  - **Superior** and **middle turbinates** are parts of **ethmoidal bone**.

Inferior Meatus

- **Nasolacrimal duct** opens into it
- Site for **maxillary antral puncture** and wash out
- Site for **intranasal antrostomy**

Middle Meatus

- Structures opening into it from anterior to posterior are:
  - **Frontal sinus** through frontonasal duct
  - **Anterior ethmoidal** cells
  - **Middle ethmoidal** cells
  - **Maxillary sinus**
- Has **bulla ethmoidalis** formed by middle ethmoidal cells
- **Hiatus seminularis** is a curved depression below the bullae

Superior Meatus

- **Posterior ethmoidal** cells open into it

Sphenoethmoidal Recess

- Lies above superior turbinate
- **Sphenoidal sinus** opens into it

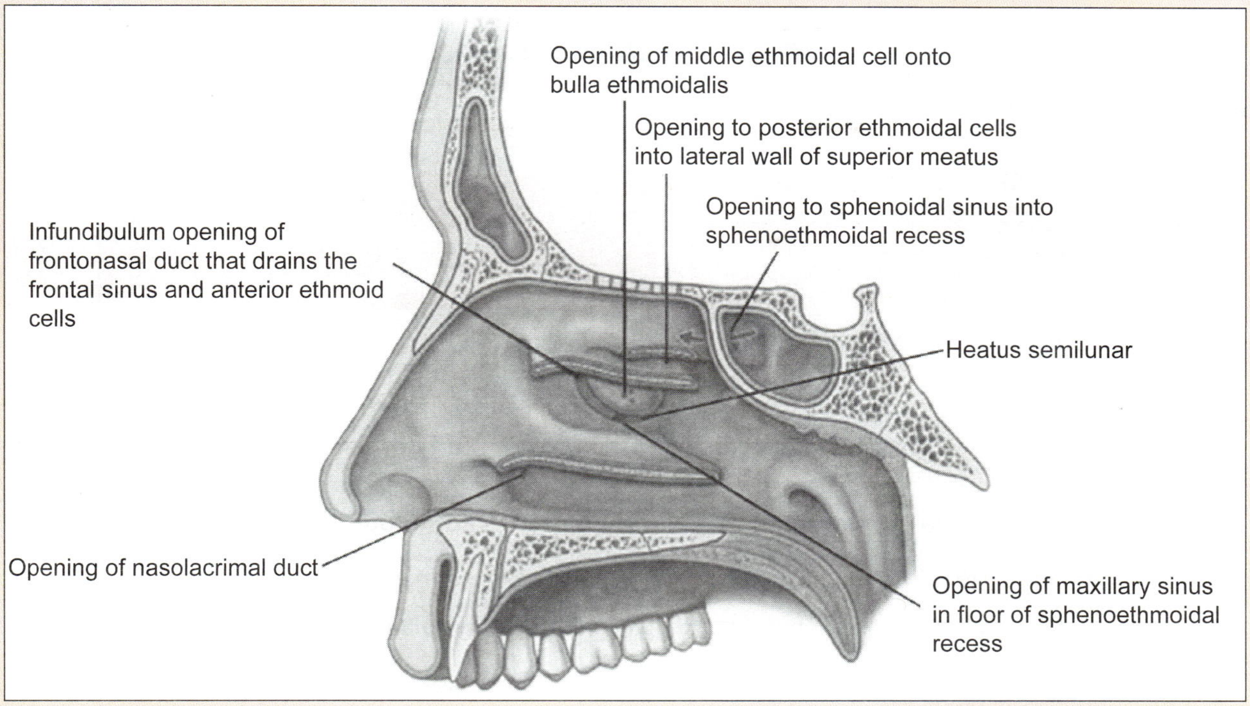

Ans: (b) Superior meatus

Ref: *Diseases of Ear, Nose and Throat by Dhingra, 5th edition, 2010, Page 76*

OPHTHALMOLOGY

1. Tigroid pattern sign in eye is seen in:

(a) Shagreen degeneration
(b) Degenerative myopia
(c) Pantothenate kinase deficiency
(d) Retinitis Pigmentosa

Explanation:

Tigroid Appearance:

- Gross tessellation of the retinal background which appears like Tiger skin (with alternate lines of black and orange)
- **Tesselation** is due to **chorioretinal degeneration** seen in **Pathological Myopia***

Pathological myopia:

- It is a rapidly progressive refractive error resulting in **high myopia (>-6 D)** and is usually associated with **degenerative changes** in the eye
- Other fundus findings are:
  - **Optic disc:** Large **pale myopic disc** with **temporal myopic crescent** and **nasal supertraction crescent**.
  - **Macula**: **Foster – Fuch's spots** and **chorio retinal atrophic patches**.
  - **Peripheral retinal degenerations** like **Lattice, Cystoid** etc will lead to **retinal hole/tear** and then **retinal detachment**.
  - **Posterior staphyloma** due to **ectasia of the sclera.**
- Vitreous liquefaction and Posterior vitreous detachment also occur.

Ans: (b) Degenerative myopia

Ref: *Kanski Clinical Ophthalmology, 8th edition, Page 632*

2. Oguchi's disease is:

(a) Retinitis Pigmentosa
(b) Fundus Albipunctatus
(c) Congenital stationary Night blindness
(d) Cone dystrophy

Explanation:

Congenital Stationary Night Blindness (CSNB)

- Refers to a group of disorders characterized by **early onset of night blindness** in the **infancy** itself but the **retinal dysfunction** is **not progressive**.
- **Types:**
  - With normal fundus.
  - With abnormal fundus – **Oguchi's disease** and **fundus albipunctatus.**
- **Oguchi's Disease:**
  - The fundus has an unusual golden-yellow colour in the light-adapted state, which becomes normal after prolonged dark adaptation. This is called **Mizuo or Mizuo-Nakamura phenomenon*.**

- Rod function is absent after 30 minutes of dark adaptation but recovers to a near-normal level after a long period of dark adaptation.
- **Fundus albipunctatus:**
  - Characterized by multiple tiny yellow spots at the posterior pole.

Ans: (c) Congenital stationary Night blindness

Ref: *Kanski Clinical Ophthalmology, 8th edition, Page 658*

3. Slow eye movement in the direction of a moving object and a rapid return of eye position in the opposite direction is known as:

(a) End gaze nystagmus
(b) Vestibular nystagmus
(c) Optokinetic nystagmus
(d) Bell's phenomenon

Explanation:

- **End gaze nystagmus, Vestibular Nystagmus and Optokinetic nystagmus are Physiological.**

OPTOKINETIC NYSTAGMUS (OKN)

- **It is a normal response when a person is fixing a moving target.**
- **Slow drifting** movement is called **smooth pursuit.**
- The **Fast jerky** correcting movement is called **saccades.**
- **Parieto-occipito temporal** region control the **slow (pursuit) phase**.
- **Frontal** lobe control the **rapid saccadic phase**.
- Uses of OKN :
  - To assess **Visual acuity** in infants
  - To rule out **malingering**
- In parieto-occipital junctional lesions, OKN will be asymmetric.

End-point Nystagmus

- It is a fine **jerk** nystagmus of **moderate frequency** seen in **extremes of gaze**.
- The fast phase is in the direction of gaze.

Vestibular Nystagmus:

- It is a **jerk nystagmus** caused by **altered input** from the **vestibular nuclei** to the **horizontal gaze centres**.

Ans: (c) Optokinetic nystagmus

Ref: *Kanski Clinical Ophthalmology, 8th edition, Page 833-834*

4. Identify the grade the hypertensive retinopathy in the fundus picture given:

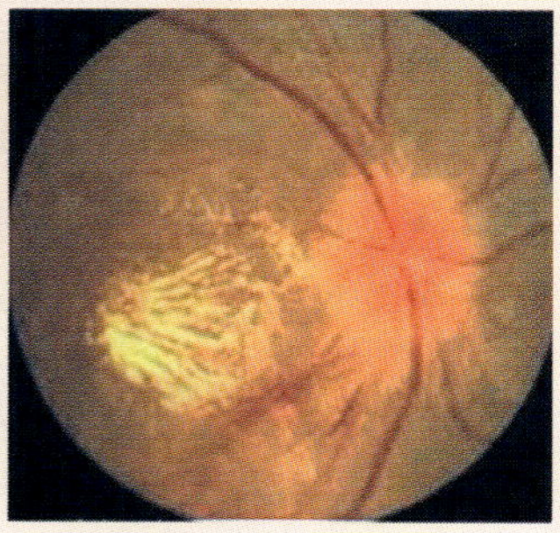

(a) Grade I HTR
(b) Grade II HTR
(c) Grade III HTR
(d) Grade IV HTR

Explanation:

- Fundus shows **silver wiring** of arterioles, **Grade III changes** and **Papilloedema** consistent with **Grade IV HTR***.

Keith Wagner and Barker Classification of Hypertensive Retinopathy (HTR)

Grades of HTR	Features in Retina
Grade - I	• Generalized arteriolar narrowing
Grade - II	• Generalized arteriolar narrowing • **Salu's Sign** – Deflection of vein at AV crossings
Grade - III	• **Copper Wiring** of arterioles • **Bonnet's Sign:** Banking of veins distal to AV crossings • **Gunn's Sign**: Tapering of veins on either side of AV crossings • Retinal hemorrhages, Cotton-wool spots and hard exudates
Grade - IV	• **Silver wiring** of arterioles + Grade III changes • **Papilloedema***

Ans: (d) Grade IV HTR

Ref: *Parson's Diseases of the Eye, 22nd edition, Page 332*

5. Identify the grade the Diabetic retinopathy given in the picture:
(a) Moderate NPDR
(b) Severe NPDR
(c) Proliferative Diabetic Retinopathy
(d) Advanced Diabetic diseases

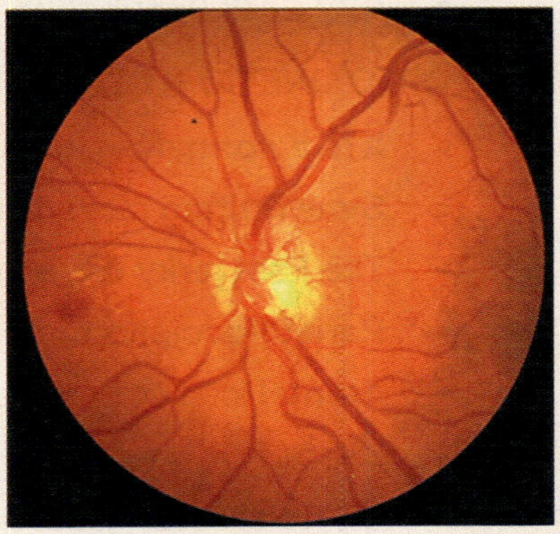

Explanation:

- The fundus picture shows **Neovascularisation** of **the disc**. So the grading of DR will be **Proliferative Diabetic retinopathy***.

Early treatment diabetic retinopathy study (ETDRS) classification

- Non-proliferative diabetic retinopathy (NPDR)
- Proliferative diabetic retinopathy (PDR)
- Diabetic Macular edema (DME)

Non-proliferative diabetic retinopathy (NPDR)

Mild	Few microaneurysms Retinal haemorrhage Hard exudates in 1 or 2 quadrants
Moderate	Above findings seen in 2 or 3 quadrants
Severe	**4:2:1 Rule** • **Haemorrhages** Or **Microaneurysms** or both In All 4 Quadrants • **Venous Beading** In 2 Quadrants • **IRMA** (**Intra Retinal Microvascular abnormality** – A-V shunts secondary to microvascular occlusion) in at least 1 Quadrant
Very severe	Any two of the above 4:2:1 rule

Proliferative diabetic retinopathy:

- Neovascularization of the Disc (NVD)
- Neovascularization elsewhere (NVE)

Advanced diabetic eye disease:

- Neovascular glaucoma
- Tractional retinal detachment

- Vitreous hemorrhage
- The treatment of PDR in this stage is **pan-retinal photocoagulation***

Ans: (c) Proliferative Diabetic Retinopathy

Ref: *A.K. Khurana's Comprehensive Ophthalmology, 7th edition, Page 311*

6. Dark choroid in FFA is seen in:

(a) Retinitis Pigmentosa
(b) Age related Macular Degeneration
(c) Leber's congenital dystrophy
(d) Stargardt's disease

Explanation:

Stargardt's Disease/Juvenile macular dystrophy

- Due to the accumulation of **lipofuscin*** within the **Retinal pigment epithelium (RPE)***.
- **Dark Choroid/Silent Choroid in FFA**–Masking of choroidal vasculature by lipofuscin accumulation in the RPE.
- Other features: **Retinal flecks***, **beaten bronze appearance*** in the **macula.**
- **ERG and EOG** is **subnormal.**
- **Fundus Flavimaculatous/Flecked retinal dystrophy: Fish tail like deep retinal flecks** are characteristic – is a subtype of **Stargardt's Disease.**

Ans: (d) Stargardt's disease

Ref: *Parson's Diseases of the Eye, 22nd edition, Page 337*

7. A 7-year-old boy is brought with complaints of defective vision in his right eye for 3 months. On examination, yellow reflex is seen in the pupillary region of right eye. On fundus examination, large, raised yellowish areas of exudation is seen in the posterior pole of the fundus. What is the most probable diagnosis?

(a) Toxocariasis
(b) Toxoplasmosis
(c) Coats' disease
(d) Incontinenta Pigmentii

Explanation:

Causes of Yellow Reflex/White Pupillary Reflex in Children

- Congenital cataract*
- Retinoblastoma*
- Retinopathy of Prematurity*
- Persistent hyperplastic primary vitreous*
- Toxocariasis*
- Coats' disease *
- Incontinenta pigmentii

Coat's Disease

- 95% unilateral
- 75% seen in boys

- Retinal arteries showing multiple aneurysms which leaks plasma into the surrounding retina in the posterior pole → **Exudative vitreoretinopathy***.

Incontinenta Pigmentii

- X-linked dominant.
- Girls are affected, male fetus are lost during pregnancy itself.
- **Retinal detachment** is the most commonly diagnosed eye finding in IP.

Toxocara

- Due to retinal invasion by **Nematode larvae Toxocara Catis and Canis** (**Round Worms**).
- **Retina:** It manifests as raised **Granuloma with tractional bands** and **Endophthalmitis.**

Ans: (c) Coats' disease

Ref: *Parson's Diseases of the Eye, 22nd edition, Page 323*

8. Drug of choice for Acanthamoeba keratitis:

(a) Dilaxanide furoate
(b) Paromomycin eye ointment
(c) Chlorhexidine
(d) Azithromycin single dose 1 gm

Explanation:

- **Acanthamoeba castellani** is a free living protozoa found in soil and fresh water.
- Risk factor – **Wearing Contact Lens***
- **Clinical features**
  - Severe pain as it causes **Keratoneuritis**
  - **Ring Abscess** is seen in cornea
- **Culture – Non-Nutrient Agar with E Coli onlay**
- **Treatment**
  - 0.02% **PHMB** (Polyhexamethyl biguanide – **Drug of choice**)
  - Others–**Neomycin**, **propamidine**, **clotrimazole**, **Chlorhexidine**
  - **Oral Ketoconazole** / **Itraconazole** 400 mg/day can also be given if the ulcer is progressing

Ans: (c) Chlorhexidine

Ref: *Parson's Diseases of the Eye, 22nd edition, Page 209*

9. Identify the marked layer in the retina:

(a) Outer plexiform layer
(b) Ganglion cell layer
(c) Inner plexiform layer
(d) Photoreceptor layer

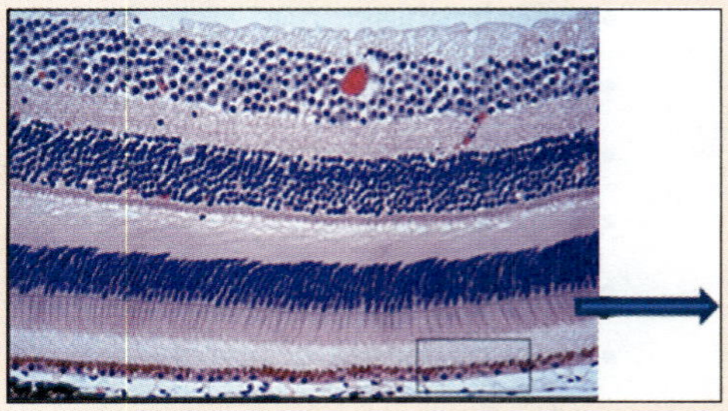

Explanation:

Ten Retinal layers: Arranged outside to inside

- Pigmented layer
- Rod and cones are projected into pigmented layer (Photoreceptor layer)

- External limiting membrane
- Outer nuclear layer
- Outer plexiform layer
- **Inner nuclear layer**
- **Inner plexiform layer**
- **Ganglionic layer**
- Nerve fiber layer
- Inner limiting membrane

ALSO NOTE:

- **Inner nuclear layer, Inner plexiform layer, Ganglionic layer and Nerve fiber layer** are absent in **Foveal region***.

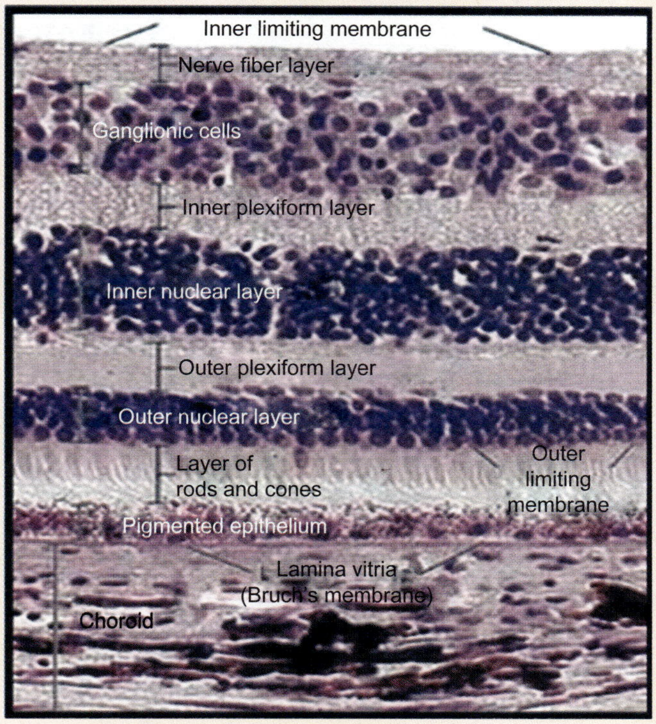

Ref: *Parson's Diseases of the Eye, 22nd edition, Page 10*

Ans: (d) Photoreceptor layer

MEDICINE

1. Pericardial knock is seen in:

(a) Cardiac tamponade
(b) Restrictive cardiomyopathy
(c) Constrictive pericarditis
(d) None of the above

Explanation:

Systolic sounds

Early systolic sounds: Aortic and pulmonary ejection sounds, closing sounds of prosthetic valves

Mid to late systolic sounds:

Non-ejection sounds or clicks

Diastolic sounds

Early diastolic sounds: Opening snaps (OS), tumor plop, pericardial knock, opening sounds of prosthetic valves

Mid diastolic sounds: S3

Late diastolic sounds: S4

Ejection click	• Sharp, High pitched sound • Audible during early systole • Seen in **Aortic stenosis, pulmonary stenosis** and **Hypertension**
Opening snap	• Brief, High pitched sound • Audible during early systole between 0.04 and 0.12 sec after A2 • Seen in **Mitral stenosis** and **Tricuspid stenosis**
Pericardial knock	• High pitched sound, heard later than OS • Audible during early diastole • Seen in **Constrictive pericarditis***
Tumor plop	• Low pitched sound • Audible during early diastole • Seen in **atrial myxoma***

Ans: (c) Constrictive pericarditis

Ref: *Harrison's Principles of Internal Medicine, 20th edition, Page 1672*

2. A chronic alcoholic presented with vomiting and proximal weakness. His ECG is shown below. Most probable diagnosis:

(a) Hypocalcemia
(b) Hypokalemia
(c) Hyperkalemia
(d) Hypercalcemia

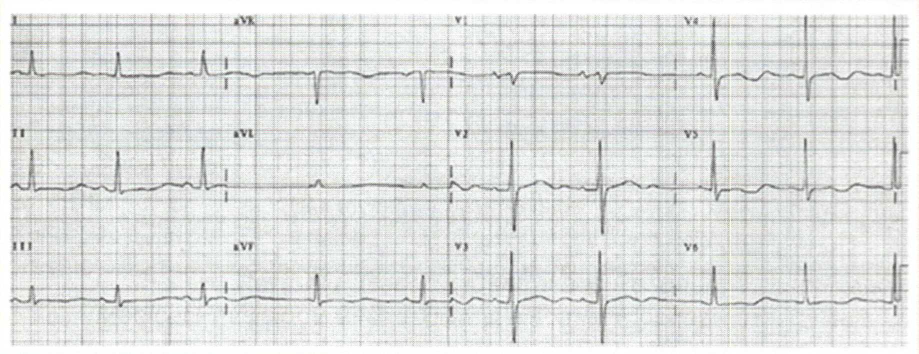

Explanation:

ECG changes in:

Hypokalemia	Hyperkalemia
• Prominent **U waves** • Nonspecific **ST depression** and **T-wave flattening** as the U wave becomes more prominent • Prolongation of the QU interval • Fusion of the T and U waves • Ventricular arrhythmias, especially torsade de pointes	• 5.5-6.5 **Tall peaked T waves (Early sign)** • 6.5-7.5 Loss of P waves • 7.0-8.0 Widening of QRS complexes • > 8.0 **Sine wave pattern***, ventricular arrhythmias, asystole
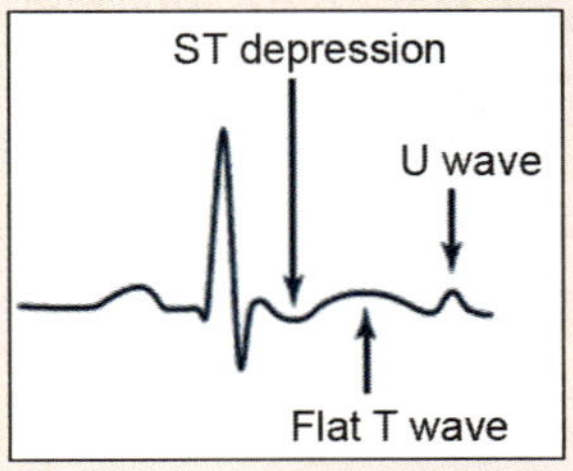	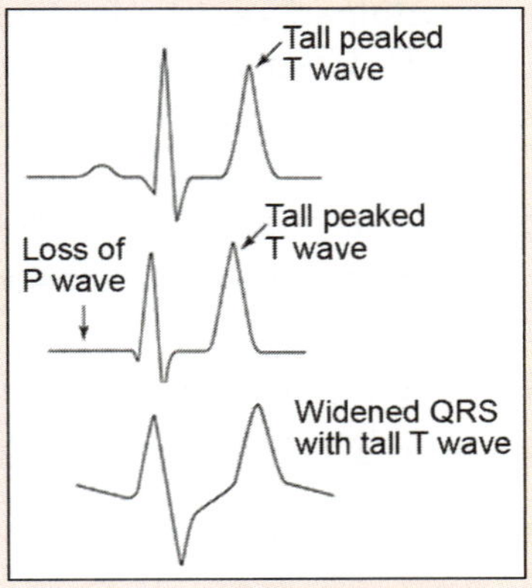

Ans: (b) Hypokalemia

Ref: *Basic and Bedside Electrocardiography by Romulo F. Baltazar, Page 406, Harrison's Principles of Internal Medicine, 20th edition, Page 31*

3. Patient admitted with acute ischemic stroke. Blood pressure should be decreased only if it is more than:

(a) 220/110 mm Hg
(b) 185/95 mm Hg
(c) 220/120 mm Hg
(d) 240/110 mm Hg

Explanation:

- When ischemic stroke occurs, the immediate goal is to optimize cerebral perfusion in the surrounding ischemic penumbra. Because collateral blood flow within the ischemic brain is blood pressure dependent blood pressure should be reduced
  - If it exceeds **220/120 mm Hg***
  - **Malignant hypertension***
  - Concomitant **myocardial ischemia***
  - If blood pressure is **>185/110** mm Hg and **thrombolytic therapy** is anticipated

Ans: (c) 220/120 mm Hg

Ref: *Harrison's Principles of Internal Medicine, 20th edition, Page 3080*

4. All the following statements are true regarding this ECG except:

(a) Seen in ischemia
(b) Seen in hypokalemia
(c) Treated with Ibutilide
(d) Can convert to ventricular fibrillation

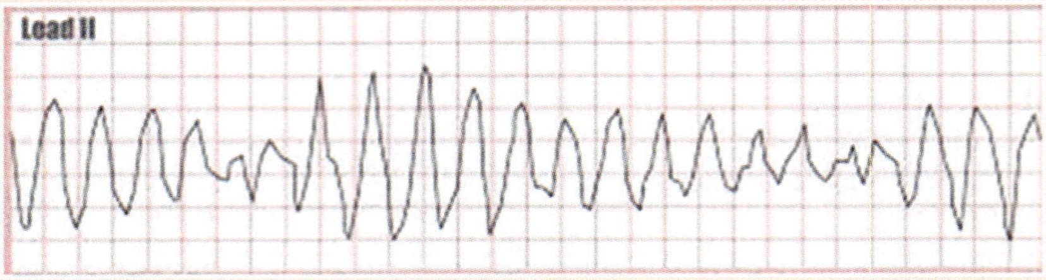

Explanation:

Ventricular tachycardia is classified based on:

Duration	Appearance (in any given lead)
• **Nonsustained ventricular tachycardia (VT):** Lasting 30 secs or less • **Sustained VT:** Longer than 30 sec in duration OR requiring direct current (DC) shock due to hemodynamic instability	• ***Monomorphic:*** All QRS complexes look the same in a given lead • ***Polymorphic:*** QRS shapes, directions, and sometimes rate vary from beat to beat

PVT with prolonged QT interval – Torsade de pointes

PVT with normal QT interval – Regular form of PVT

I. With QT(U) prolongation (torsade de pointes)

A. Hereditary (congenital) long QT syndrome
B. Acquired long QT syndrome
  (1) Drug-induced:
    Cardiac agents (e.g., quinidine, sotalol, ibutilide, dofetilide)
    Non-cardiac agents (e.g., tricyclic antidepressants, methadone, haloperidol)
  (2) Metabolic (e.g., hypokalemia, hypomagnesemia)
  (3) Bradyarrhythmias (esp. high-degree atrioventricular block)
  (4) Other (e.g., subarachnoid hemorrhage)

II. Without QT(U) prolongation

A. Acute ischemia
B. "Channelopathies"
  (1) Catecholaminergic polymorphic ventricular tachycardia (CPVT)
  (2) Brugada syndrome
  (3) Short QT syndrome

III. Bidirectional ventricular tachycardia

A. Digitalis toxicity
B. CPVT

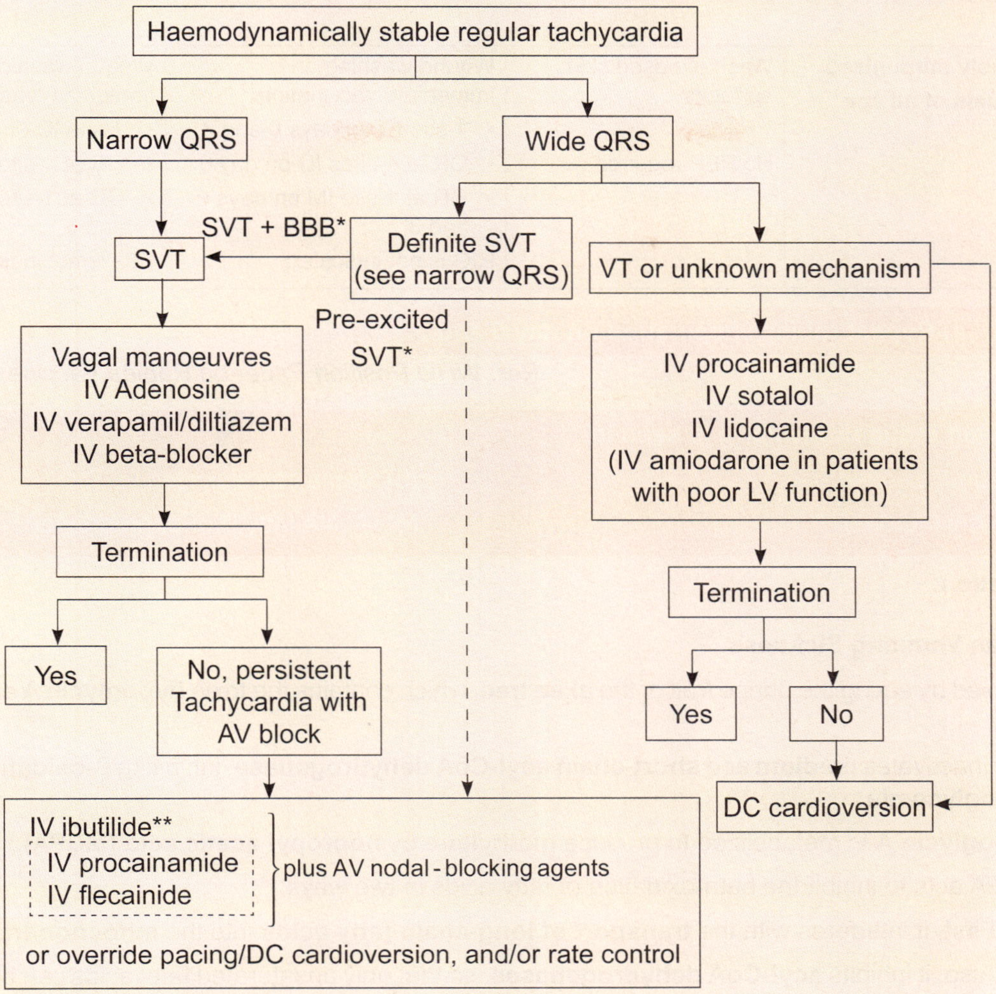

Ans: (c) Treated with Ibutilide

Ref: *Goldberger's Clinical Electrocardiography: A Simplified Approach, 9th edition, Page 166; The ESC Textbook of Intensive and Acute Cardiovascular Care, 2nd edition, Page 518*

5. A patient who has got complete anti rabies vaccination 2 years ago was bitten by a dog and he is bleeding. What should you do now?

(a) Repeat rabies vaccination on day 0 and 3
(b) Give only anti rabies immunoglobulin
(c) Repeat full vaccine schedule
(d) No vaccination is warranted

Explanation:

	Category I exposure	Category II exposure	Category III exposure
Immunologically Naive individuals of all age groups	Wash exposed skin surfaces No PEP required	Wound washing and immediate vaccination: • 2-sites ID on days 0, 3 and 7 • OR 1-site IM on days 0, 3, 7 and between day 14 and 28 • OR 2-sites IM on days 0 and 1-site IM on days 7, 21 RIG is not indicated.	Wound washing and immediate vaccination • 2-sites ID on days 0, 3 and 7 • OR 1-site IM on days 0, 3, 7 and between day 14 and 28 • OR 2-sites IM on days 0 and 1-site IM on days 7, 21 RIG administration is recommended.

Contd.

Contd.

Previously immunized individuals of all age groups	Wash exposed skin surfaces No PEP required	Wound washing and immediate vaccination: • 1-site ID on days 0 and 3 • OR at 4-sites ID on day 0 • OR at 1-site IM on days 0 and 3 RIG is not indicated.	Wound washing and immediate vaccination: • 1-site ID on days 0 and 3 • OR at 4-sites ID on day 0 • OR at 1-site IM on days 0 and 3 RIG is not indicated.

Ans: (a) Repeat rabies vaccination on day 0 and 3

Ref: *WHO Position Paper on Rabies Vaccine, February 2018*

6. Hypoglycin induced vomiting is seen in:

(a) Refsums disease
(b) Jamaican sickness
(c) Reyes syndrome
(d) Acute fatty liver of pregnancy

Explanation:

Jamaican Vomiting Sickness

- Caused by eating the unripe fruit of the **akee tree**, which contains the toxin **hypoglycin A and Hypoglycin B.**
- This inactivates **medium** and **short-chain acyl-CoA dehydrogenase,** inhibiting **β-oxidation** and causing **hypoglycemia.**
- **Hypoglycin A** is metabolized to produce **methylene cyclopropyl acetic acid (MCPA).**
- MCPA acts to inhibit the beta-oxidation of fatty acids in two ways:
  - First, it interferes with the **transport of long-chain fatty acids** into the **mitochondria.**
  - Also, it inhibits **acyl-CoA dehydrogenases,** so that only unsaturated fatty acids can be fully oxidized.
- Fatty acids accumulate in the liver in a **microvesicular pattern*** that can be seen on biopsy.

Ans: (b) Jamaican sickness

Ref: *Harpers Illustrated Biochemistry, 31st edition, Page 532*

7. In JVP, Y descent absent in:

(a) Restrictive cardiomyopathy
(b) Severe tricuspid regurgitation
(c) Constrictive pericarditis
(d) Cardiac tamponade

Explanation:

Waveforms in JVP

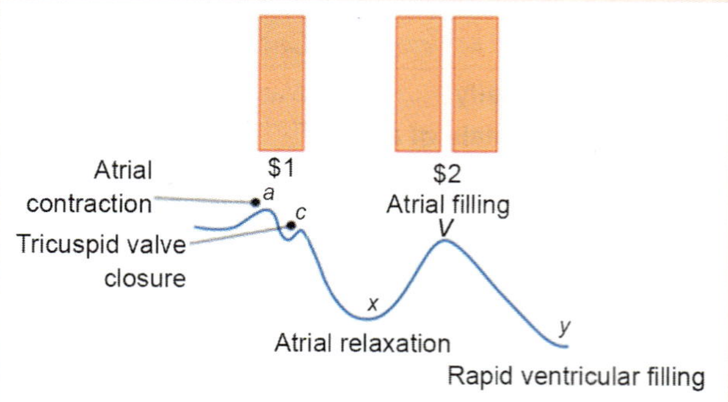

Abnormal α waves

Large α waves	Cannon waves	Absent α waves
• TS, RA myxomas, tricuspid atresia • PH, PS, acute PE • RV cardiomyopathy • RV infarction • Severe AS, HCM	• Junctional rhythm VT 1:1 retrograde conduction • Iso rhythmic AV dissociation • CHB, VT, VPC, classic AV dissociation, ventricular pacing	• Atrial fibrillation

Abnormal *x* descent

Prominent *x* descent	Absent *x* descent
• Constrictive pericarditis • Cardiac tamponade • Atrial septal defect	• Tricuspid regurgitation (TR)

Abnormal *v* waves

Prominent *v* waves	Diminished *v* waves
• Tricuspid regurgitation (TR) • Large atrial septal defect • Gerbode's defect • Severe congestive heart failure • Corpulmonale	• Hypovolemia • Use of nitrates

Abnormal *y* descent

Rapid *y* descent	Slow *y* descent
• Severe tricuspid regurgitation • Constrictive pericarditis • Restrictive cardiomyopathy	• Tricuspid stenosis • Right atrial myxoma • Cardiac tamponade

Ans: (d) Cardiac tamponade

Ref: *Hursts The Heart, 14th edition, Page 236*

8. A case of monkey bite with deep 2*2 cm abrasion over the face. What should you do?

(a) Antibiotics + consider acyclovir for macaca monkey bites
(b) Antibiotics and rabies vaccination
(c) Topical antibiotics
(d) Wound washing and antibiotics

Explanation:

- Bites from **Old World monkeys *(Macaca)*** result in the transmission of **B virus *(Macacine herpesvirus 1, Herpesvirus simiae, Cercopithecine herpesvirus),*** a cause of serious infection of the human central nervous system

Biting species	Commonly isolated pathogens	Preferred antibiotic(s)	Alternative in penicillin-allergic patient	Prophylaxis advised	Other considerations
Dog	*Staphylococcus aureus, Pasteurella multocida, anaerobes, Capnocytophaga canimorsus*	Amoxicillin/clavulanate (250–500 mg PO tid) or ampicillin/sulbactam (1.5–3.0 g IV q6h)	Clindamycin (150–300 mg PO qid) plus either TMP-SMX (1 DS tablet PO bid) or ciprofloxacin (500 mg PO bid)	Sometimes	Consider rabies prophylaxis

Contd.

Contd.

Cat	*P. multocida, S. aureus,* anaerobes	Amoxicillin/ clavulanate or ampicillin/sulbactam	Clindamycin plus TMP-SMX or fluoroquinolone	Usually	Consider rabies prophylaxis
Human, occlusional	Viridans streptococci, *S. aureus, Haemophilus influenzae, anaerobes*	Amoxicillin/ clavulanate or ampicillin/sulbactam	Erythromycin (500 mg PO qid) or fluoroquinolone	Always	
Human, clenched-fist	As for occlusional, plus *Eikenella corrodens*	Ampicillin/ sulbactam or imipenem (500 mg q6h)	Cefoxitin	Always	Examine for tendon, nerve, or joint involvement
Monkey	As for human bite	As for human bite	As for human bite	Always	For macaque monkeys, consider B virus prophylaxis with acyclovir
Snake	*Pseudomonas aeruginosa, Proteus* spp., *Bacteroides fragilis, Clostridium* spp.	Ampicillin/ sulbactam	Clindamycin plus TMP-SMX or fluoroquinolone	Sometimes, especially with venomous snakes	Administer antivenin for venomous snakebite
Rodent	*Streptobacillus moniliformis, Leptospira* spp., *P. multocida*	Penicillin VK (500 mg PO qid)	Doxycycline (100 mg PO bid)	Sometimes	

Ans: (a) Antibiotics + consider acyclovir for macaca monkey bites

Ref: *Harrison's Principles of Internal Medicine, 20th edition, Page 1019*

9. A patient with alcoholic cirrhosis has a MELD score of 20-29. What is the percentage of mortality in next 3 months?

(a) 2% (b) 19.6%

(c) 52.3% (d) 25%

Explanation:

3-Month Mortality Based on MELD Score

MELD Score	Mortality Probability
40	71.3% mortality
30-39	52.6% mortality
20-29	19.6% mortality
10-19	6.0% mortality
9 or less	1.9% mortality

Ans: (b) 19.6%

Ref: *Sleisenger and Fordtran's Gastrointestinal and Liver Disease, 10th edition, Page 1630*

10. A 45 years male has active calcium oxalate nephrolithiasis. His blood pressure was not controlled by dietary and exercise modifications. What will you give now?

(a) Losartan (b) Chlorthalidone

(c) Furosemide (d) Atenolol

Explanation:

- A thiazide diuretic, in doses higher than those used to treat **hypertension, lower urine calcium excretion.**
- Several randomized controlled trials have demonstrated that **thiazide diuretics,** most commonly **chlorthalidone,** can reduce **calcium oxalate** stone recurrence by **~50%.**

Ans: (b) Chlorthalidone

Ref: *Harrison's Principles of Internal Medicine, 20th edition, Page 2172*

11. A patient with postpartum hemorrhage had about 2 liters of blood loss. Investigation revealed normal PT and a prolonged aPTT. Test to differentiate between coagulation factor deficiency and factor inhibitor is:

(a) Tissue thromboplastin inhibition time
(b) Ecarin clotting time
(c) Dilute Russel viper venom time
(d) Mixing studies

Explanation:

- **Mixing studies** are used to evaluate a **prolonged aPTT or, less commonly PT,** to distinguish between a factor deficiency and an **inhibitor.**

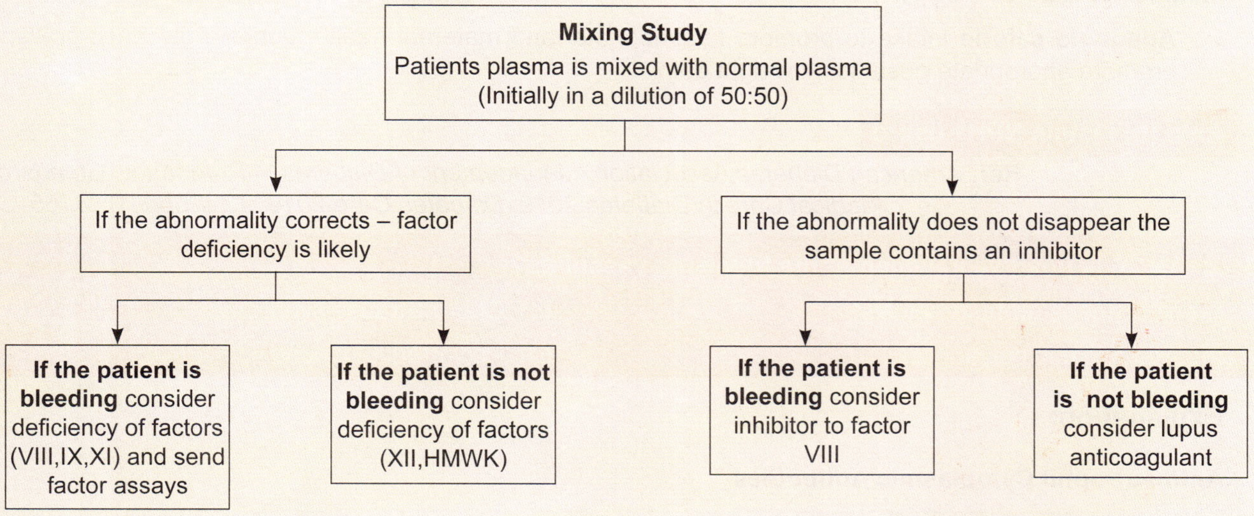

Ans: (d) Mixing studies

Ref: *Harrison's Principles of Internal Medicine, 20th edition, Page 410*

12. Most physiological insulin during pregnancy:

(a) Insulin regular+NPH
(b) Insulin NPH+lispro
(c) Insulin degludec
(d) Insulin lispro+insulin regular

Explanation:

- **Management of Pre-existing Type 1 Diabetes and Type 2 Diabetes in Pregnancy**

Insulin Use – Recommendation

- Early in the first trimester, there is an increase in insulin requirements, followed by a decrease in **weeks 9 through 16 weeks.**
- After **16 weeks,** rapidly increasing insulin resistance requires weekly increases in insulin dose.
- *In general, a smaller proportion of the total daily dose should be given as* ***basal insulin*** *(50%) and a* ***greater proportion (50%) as prandial insulin.***

Glycemic Targets in Pregnancy:

- **Fasting** and **postprandial self-monitoring** of blood glucose are recommended

- HbA1c Target is 6%.
- Pregnancy is a low glucose state.
- **ADA-recommended targets** for women with **type 1** or **type 2 diabetes** are as follows:
  - Fasting **– 95 mg/dL (5.3 mmol/L)** and either
  - One-hour postprandial – **140 mg/dL (7.8 mmol/L)** OR
  - Two-hour postprandial – **120 mg/dL (6.7 mmol/L)**

MANAGEMENT OF GESTATIONAL DIABETES MELLITUS

Recommendations

- **Lifestyle change** is an essential component of management of gestational diabetes mellitus.
- **Insulin** is the preferred medication as it **does not cross** the placenta.

LIFESTYLE MANAGEMENT

Medical Nutrition Therapy

- **Adequate calorie** intake to promote fetal/neonatal and maternal health, achieve glycemic goals, and promote appropriate gestational weight gain.

Ans: (b) Insulin NPH+ lispro

Ref: *American Diabetes Association, Management of Diabetes in Pregnancy: Standards of Medical Care in Diabetes 2019, Diabetes Care 2019; 42 (Suppl.1): S165–S172*

13. c- ANCA is positive in which of the following vasculitis?

(a) Wegener's granulomatosis (b) Churg-Strauss syndrome
(c) Microscopic polyangiitis (d) Polyarteritis nodosa

Explanation:

Antineutrophil Cytoplasmic Antibodies

Antibody	pANCA	cANCA
	• Localized perinuclear or nuclear staining pattern of the indicator neutrophils	• 29-kDa neutral serine proteinase present in neutrophil azurophilic granules
Major target antigen	• **Myeloperoxidase**	• **Proteinase-3**
Other possible antigens	• **Elastase, cathepsin G, lactoferrin, lysozyme and bactericidal/ permeability-increasing protein Proteinase-3**	
Diseases	• **Microscopic polyangiitis, eosinophilic** granulomatosis with polyangiitis **(Churg-Strauss syndrome)** • **Isolated necrotizing crescentic glomerulonephritis** • Granulomatosis with polyangiitis **(Wegener's)**	• **Wegener's granulomatosis** (Granulomatosis with polyangiitis)

Ans: (a) Wegener's granulomatosis

Ref: *Harrison's Principles of Internal Medicine, 20th edition, Page 2575*

14. A 20 years female had dogbite. Now she has fever, vomiting and diarrhea. The probable causative agent for this condition is:

(a) Porphyromon gingivalis (b) Selenomonac
(c) Capnocytophaga (d) Veilonella

Explanation:

- Capnocytophaga canimorsus is a bacterial cause of fulminant sepsis among individuals who have been bitten by a dog.
- Clinical features include fever, vomiting, diarrhea, abdominal pain, hypotension, chest pain, bleeding from gums, hematuria, headache, meningeal signs.
- ***C. canimorsus*** causes a wide range of infections, including **severe sepsis** with **shock** and **disseminated intravascular coagulation, meningitis, endocarditis, cellulitis and septic arthritis.**

Capnocytophaga Species

- This genus of **fastidious, fusiform, gram-negative coccobacilli** is **facultatively anaerobic** and requires an atmosphere enriched in carbon dioxide for optimal growth.
- ***C. ochracea, C. gingivalis and C. sputigena*** have been associated with **sepsis** in **immunocompromised hosts,** particularly **neutropenic patients** with **hematologic malignancy,** and probably play a role in localized **juvenile periodontitis** in the immunocompetent host.
- ***C. canimorsus and C. cynodegmi*** *are endogenous to the* ***canine mouth.*** *Patients infected with these species frequently have a history of* ***dog bites*** *or of* ***exposure to dogs*** *without scratches or bites.*

Treatment:

- **Clindamycin** (600–900 mg every 6–8 h).
- Penicillin derivative plus a Beta-lactamase inhibitor—such as **ampicillin/sulbactam** (1.5–3.0 g of ampicillin every 6 h)—are currently recommended for empirical treatment of infections caused by **C. ochracea, C. gingivalis and C. sputigena.**
- Infections with **C. canimorsus** should be treated with **penicillin** (12–18 million units every 4 h). This regimen or ampicillin/sulbactam should be given prophylactically to asplenic patients sustaining dog-bite injuries.
- C. canimorsus is also susceptible to **clindamycin, imipenem, fluoroquinolones,** and third-generation **cephalosporins.**

Ans: (c) Capnocytophaga

Ref: *Harrison's Infectious Diseases,1st edition, Page 479*

15. Statin induced myopathy is seen more commonly among:

(a) Elderly (b) End stage renal disease
(c) Hepatic disorders (d) Children

Explanation:

"CKD is a common **risk factor** for the development of **statin-induced myopathy".**

Other risk factors are:

- Pre existing neuromuscular diseases
- Hypothyroidism
- Hypovitaminosis D
- Concurrent usage or drugs–Steroids, Cyclosporine, Zidovudine, Daptomycin

Myopathy from Lipid-Lowering Agents

- All classes of lipid-lowering agents have been implicated in muscle toxicity, including:
  - **Fibrates** (clofibrate, gemfibrozil)
  - **HMG-CoA reductase inhibitors *(statins)***
  - **Niacin** (nicotinic acid)
  - **Ezetimibe**
- Myalgia, malaise and muscle tenderness are the most common manifestations.
- Patients may exhibit **proximal weakness.** Varying degrees of **muscle necrosis** are seen, and in severe reactions **rhabdomyolysis** and **myoglobinuria** occur.
- Concomitant use of **statins with fibrates** and **cyclosporine** is more likely to cause adverse reactions than use of one agent alone.
- Elevated **serum CK** is an important indication of toxicity.
- Muscle weakness is accompanied by a **myopathic EMG,** and **muscle necrosis** is observed by muscle biopsy.

Ans: (b) End stage renal disease

Ref: *Harrison's Principles of Internal Medicine, 20th edition, Page 3253*

16. Microangiopathic hemolytic anemia (MAHA) is seen in all conditions except:

(a) TTP (b) PNH

(c) Cardiac prosthetic valves (d) DIC

Explanation:

- **Microangiopathic hemolytic anemia (MAHA)** is now used to designate any **hemolytic anemia** related to **RBC fragmentation,** occurring in association with **small vessel disease**
- Hallmark is **schistocytes (Burr cells, Helmet cells, Triangle cells)** in peripheral smear
- Arterioles are changed by deposition of **platelets** and **fibrin**
- **Microvascular lesion** can even cause organ damage
- **Thrombocytopenia** occurs due to consumption of platelets

Causes:

- **TTP/HUS***
- **DIC***
- **Malignant Hypertension***
- **Eclampsia***
- **HELLP Syndrome***
- Vasculitis
- Prosthetic valves
- Transplant rejection
- Glomerulonephritis
- PAN
- Rocky Mountain Spotted Fever
- Wegener's Granulomatosis
- Burns
- SLE

- Scleroderma
- Drugs–Ciclosporine, Gemcitabine, Mitomycin C

Ans: (b) PNH

Ref: *Harrison's Principle of Internal Medicine, 20th edition, Page 708*

17. Acute leukemia in pregnancy. What should be the correct treatment plan?

(a) ATRA in first trimester
(b) Gemtuzumab-Ozagamycin
(c) ATRA in second trimester
(d) Methotrexate therapy

Explanation:

Pregnancy may affect drug metabolism due to:

- Altered distribution due to an often greatly increased plasma volume
- Presence of the amniotic sac creating a third space
- Changes in both hepatic and renal metabolism.

Drugs contraindicated in pregnancy

- Cytarabine
- Anthracycline
- Leukapheresis
- Arsenic trioxide
- Gemtuzumab Ozagamicin

Drugs which is safer

- Daunorubicin is safer
- **ATRA** if given between **3 and 5 weeks** of gestation is associated with a high incidence of fetal malformation
- The **European Leukaemia Net** recommends avoidance of **ATRA** in the **first trimester**
- **ATRA** can be introduced in the **second trimester**

Ans: (c) ATRA in second trimester

Ref: *American Society of Hematology Blood 2014 Journal: How I Treat Leukemia During Pregnancy*

18. A 55-year-old female patient had a trauma to the abdomen while encountered during an RTA. Following which she underwent a laparotomy. After a month of surgery she was admitted with fever, cough and breathlessness. She was admitted to hospital and her blood culture was sent. What could be the probable organism identified in the culture?

(a) Staphylococcus
(b) E.coli
(c) Pneumococcus
(d) Klebsiella

Explanation:

- The spleen is an organ that removes damaged red blood cells from the bloodstream.
- It also protects the body against bloodstream infection by removing bacteria from the blood.
- Splenectomised patients can have various infections due to few organisms.

Immunizations

- The following vaccines **should be given at least two weeks before** planned surgical removal of the spleen.

- The vaccine should be given **14 or more days after emergency removal of the spleen.**

Pneumococcal Vaccine

- Two types of pneumococcal vaccines are available–**PPSV23 and PCV13**.
- Young children receive PCV13 as part of their routine infant immunizations.
- PCV13 is also recommended for adults who do not have a functional spleen.
- PPSV23 is recommended for adults and children ≥2 years who do not have a functional spleen.
- PPSV23 is given at least eight weeks after PCV13 immunization.

Hib Vaccine

- Most adults have been exposed to Hib and are therefore immune.
- Experts advise people without a functional spleen to have the Hib vaccine if it was not given previously.

Meningococcal Vaccine

- A meningococcal conjugate vaccine (MCV4; Menactra or Menveo).
- A meningococcal serogroup B vaccine (Trumenba or Bexsero).

Influenza Vaccine

- Once-yearly influenza vaccination is recommended for people without a functional spleen.

Preventive Antibiotic Therapy

- Antibiotics are recommended in some people without a functional spleen to reduce the risk of developing sepsis.
- Two approaches are common:
  - Daily preventive antibiotic therapy.
  - Antibiotic therapy for fever when needed.

Ans: (c) Pneumococcus

Ref: *American Academy of Pediatrics, Pneumococcal Infections. In: Red Book: 2015 Report of the Committee on Infectious Diseases, 30th edition, Kimberlin DW, Brady MT, Jackson MA, Long SS (Eds), American Academy of Pediatrics, Elk Grove Village, IL 2015, Page 626*

19. A person developed gas gangrene due to Clostridium tetani. What is the correct treatment?

(a) Vancomycine/Metronidazole (b) Clindamycin
(c) Colistin (d) Levofloxacin

Explanation:

- **C. perfringens** is the most common of the **clostridial species** isolated from **tissue infections** and **bacteremias.**
- Next in frequency are **C. novyi and C. septicum.**

Enteritis Necroticans

- Necrotizing enteritis **(enteritis necroticans or pigbel)** is caused by β toxin produced by type C strains of C. perfringens after ingestion of a high-protein meal in conjunction with trypsin inhibitors.
- Clinical features of pigbel include:
  - Acute abdominal pain
  - Bloody diarrhea

- Vomiting
- Shock

Suppurative Deep-Tissue Infections

- These include:
  - Intraabdominal sepsis
  - Empyema, pelvic abscess
  - Subcutaneous abscess
  - Frostbite with gas gangrene
- **C. ramosum, C. perfringens and C. bifermentans** are the most commonly isolated species

Gas Gangrene (Clostridial Myonecrosis)

- Gas gangrene is characterized by:
  - Rapid and extensive necrosis of muscle
  - Gas formation and systemic toxicity
- The infection originates in a wound contaminated with clostridia.
- Gas gangrene can follow **trauma, surgery, or IM injection.**
- The wound must be deep, necrotic, and without communication to the surface.
- Gram's staining of the wound exudate shows many **gram-positive rods** with **relatively few inflammatory cells.**

Treatment of Clostridial Infections[a]

Condition	Antibiotic Treatment	Penicillin Allergy	Adjunctive Treatment/Note
Contamination	None	–	–
Gas gangrene	Penicillin, 3-4 million units IV q4h, *plus* Clindamycin, 600 mg IV q6h	Chloramphenicol, metronidazole, imipenem, doxycycline (see text)[b]	Surgical debridement with wide excision is essential. Consider hyperbaric oxygen
Clostridial sepsis	Penicillin, 3-4 million units IV q4h, *plus* Clindamycin, 600 mg IV q6h	Chloramphenicol, metronidazole, imipenem, doxycycline (see text)[b]	Transient bacteremia may be clinically insignificant
Suppurative deep-tissue infections (e.g., abdominal wall, gynecologic)	Penicillin, 3-4 million units IV q4h, plus Gentamicin, 5 mg/kg IV q24h, *OR* A third-generation cephalosporin (e.g., ceftriaxone, 2 g IV q12h)	As above, plus gentamicin or a quinolone	Empirical therapy should be given. Therapy should be based on Gram's stain and culture results when available

[a]Treatment recommendations for *C. difficile* colitis, tetanus, and botulism are found in Chaps. 43, 40 and 41, respectively
[b]Perform sensitivity testing; consider desensitization.

Ans: (a) Vancomycin/Metronidazole

Ref: *Harrison's Infectious Diseases, 1st edition, Page 440*

20. All are true regarding ventilator associated pneumonia except:

(a) Mechanical ventilation for 24 hours
(b) Hospital admission for 4 days
(c) Mechanical ventilation for at least 3 days
(d) BAL culture >10 CFU/ml

Explanation:

VENTILATOR ASSOCIATED PNEUMONIA (VAP)

Definition:

- A pneumonia where the patient is **on mechanical ventilation** for **>2 calendar days** on the date of event, with day of **ventilator placement being Day 1,***

  AND

  The ventilator was in place on the date of event or the day before.

  *If the ventilator was in place prior to inpatient admission, the ventilator day count begins with the admission date to the first inpatient location.
- Patients with severe hospital-acquired pneumonia who require mechanical ventilation after the onset of infection do not meet the definition of VAP.

Clinical Presentation

- Most patients with VAP present with a gradual or sudden onset of the following:
  - **Symptoms** – Dyspnea (few patients have symptoms since most are nonverbal on mechanical ventilation)
  - **Signs –** Fever, tachypnea, increased or purulent secretions, hemoptysis, rhonchi, crackles, reduced breath sounds, bronchospasm
  - **Ventilator mechanics –** Reduced tidal volume, increased inspiratory pressures
  - **Laboratory findings –** Worsening hypoxemia, leukocytosis
  - **Imaging –** New or progressive infiltrate on chest radiograph or computed tomography
- VAP is supported when an established threshold of bacterial growth is exceeded
- Typical thresholds include the following:
  - **Endotracheal aspirates –** ≥1,000,000 colony forming units (CFU)/mL
  - **Bronchoscopic-** or mini-BAL – 10,000 CFU/mL
  - **PSB –** 1000 CFU/mL
- **Treatment of VAP** (Any of these drugs intravenously)
  - Piperacillin-Tazobactam 4.5 gm 6th hourly
  - Cefipime 2 gm 8th hourly
  - Levofloxacin 750 mg once daily
  - Imipenem 500 mg 6th hourly
  - Meropenem 1 gm 8th hourly

Ans: (c) Mechanical ventilation for atleast 3 days

Ref: *VAP CDC Guidelines, 2019 and CMDT 2019, Page 284*

21. A 50-year-old patient has carcinoid tumor associated diarrhea and vomiting. What treatment will you give?

(a) Loperamide 3-4 hourly
(b) Octrotide S/C 20 mg three weekly/daily
(c) Octreotide 1000 mcg daily
(d) Octreotide LAR

Explanation:

- **Metastatic NETs (carcinoids)** in the **liver** frequently present as **hepatomegaly** in a patient who may have minimal symptoms and nearly **normal liver function test results**.

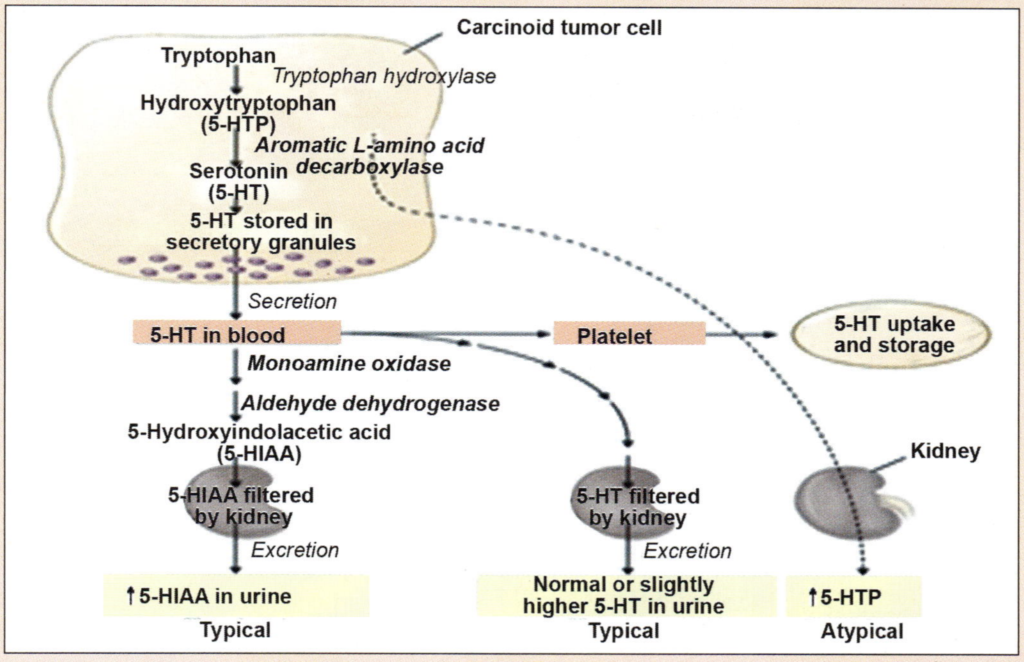

CARCINOID SYNDROME

Clinical Features

- **Flushing** and **diarrhea** are the two most common symptoms
- The diarrhea usually is described as **watery**
- Abdominal pain may be present
- Cardiac manifestations include **Pulmonary stenosis and Tricuspid regurgitation**

Treatment

- Dietary supplementation with **nicotinamide**
- Treatment of **heart failure** with **diuretics**
- Treatment of **wheezing** with **oral bronchodilators**
- Control of the diarrhea with antidiarrheal agents such as **loperamide and diphenoxylate**
- Synthetic analogues of **somatostatin (octreotide, lanreotide)**
- These drugs are effective at relieving symptoms and decreasing urinary 5-HIAA levels in patients with this syndrome
- **Octreotide-LAR (10–30 mg I.M., monthly)**
- **Lanreotide-SR/autogel (Somatuline) (60–120 mg SC-deep, monthly)**
- Octreotide-LAR (30 mg/month) gives a plasma level ≥1 ng/mL for 25 days, whereas this requires 3–6 injections a day of the non-sustained-release form
- Lanreotide-autogel (Somatuline) is given every 4–6 weeks
- **Pasireotide (SOM230)** is a somatostatin analogue with broader selectivity (high-affinity somatostatin receptors [sst1, sst2, sst3, sst5]) than octreotide/lanreotide (sst2, sst5).

Ans: (d) Octreotide LAR

Ref: *Harrison's Principles of Internal Medicine, 20th edition, Page 596*

22. Drug of choice for resistant macrophage activation syndrome:

(a) Tacrolimus
(b) Methylprednisolone
(c) Cyclosporine
(d) Tocilizumab

Explanation:

- **HLH** is an aggressive and potentially fatal syndrome that results from **inappropriate prolonged activation of lymphocytes and macrophages.**

Macrophage Activation Syndrome

- Similar to classic HLH, macrophage activation is characterized by proliferation of macrophages and T cells.
- Patients present with continuous fever, purpura, hepatosplenomegaly, mental status changes, cytopenias, coagulopathy and hypofibrinogenemia.
- Laboratory findings may include defective NK cell function and low perforin expression, as seen in HLH.
- Treatment with dexamethasone and etoposide therapy is recommended if patients fail to improve after a brief trial of therapy appropriate for rheumatologic disease.

Treatment

- Induction therapy based on the **HLH-94 protocol** consists of a series of weekly treatments with dexamethasone and etoposide (VP-16).
- Intrathecal methotrexate and hydrocortisone are given to those with central nervous system disease.
- **Etoposide (VP-16)** is given at a dose of 150 mg/m^2 is given twice weekly for the first two weeks, and once weekly for weeks three through eight.
- **Dexamethasone** is the preferred corticosteroid because it can cross the blood-brain barrier.
- Dexamethasone is given intravenously or orally and tapered over the eight-week induction:
  - Weeks 1 and 2 – 10 mg/m^2 daily
  - Weeks 3 and 4 – 5 mg/m^2 daily
  - Weeks 5 and 6 – 2.5 mg/m^2 daily
  - Week 7 – 1.25 mg/m^2 daily
  - Week 8 – Taper dose to zero
- The HLH-94 protocol also used **cyclosporin starting at week nine** (6 mg/kg daily in divided doses; target trough level 200 mcg/L).
- The major modifications of the HLH-2004 protocol were to begin cyclosporin simultaneously with etoposide and to add hydrocortisone to the intrathecal methotrexate.

REFRACTORY OR RECURRENT DISEASE

General Approach

- A relapse is typically signaled by
  - The development of fever
  - Organomegaly
  - Increasing ferritin, D-dimer, and liver enzymes
  - Falling hemoglobin and platelet levels.
- Our general approach to the treatment of patients with refractory or recurrent disease is as follows:
  - Patients who initially have disease remission with HLH-94-based therapy-retreatment using the same regimen.

- If disease worsens during induction therapy–re-escalate the doses of these agents to full dose.
- Use additional agents if there is clinical deterioration despite maximum doses of etoposide and dexamethasone.

OR

- If there is no sign of clinical improvement after the first two to three weeks of treatment.
- Our first choice is **alemtuzumab,** a monoclonal antibody to the CD52 protein expressed on the surface of mature T cells and possibly NK cells.
- **Tocilizumab** is a medicine that blocks one of the cytokines that is elevated in patients with HLH.

Clinical Criteria for Diagnosis of Hemophagocytic Lymphohistiocytosis
Hemophagocytic lymphohistiocytosis (HLH) diagnosis is established with at least five of the following: • Fever • Splenomegaly • Cytopenias in at least two cell lines: Hemoglobin <90 g/L Platelets < 100 × 10^9L Neutrophils < 1 × 10^9L • Hypertriglyceridemia and/or hypofibrinogenemia: Fasting triglycerides > 3 mmol/L (> 265 mg/dL) Fibrinogen < 1.5 g/L • Hemophagocytosis in marrow or spleen or lymph nodes • Low or absent activity of natural killer cells (specialized laboratory test) • Ferritin > 500 mcg/L (> 2000 mcg/L may be more specific) • Soluble CD 25 (soluble interleukin-2 receptor) > 2400 U/mL *OR* • HLH-associated gene mutations

Ans: (d) Tocilizumab

Ref: *Williams Hematology, 9th edition, Page 1114*

23. False regarding restrictive lung disease:

(a) FEV-1/FVC decreased (b) FVC decreased

(c) TLC decreased (d) FeV1 increased

Explanation:

How to interpret Spirometry?

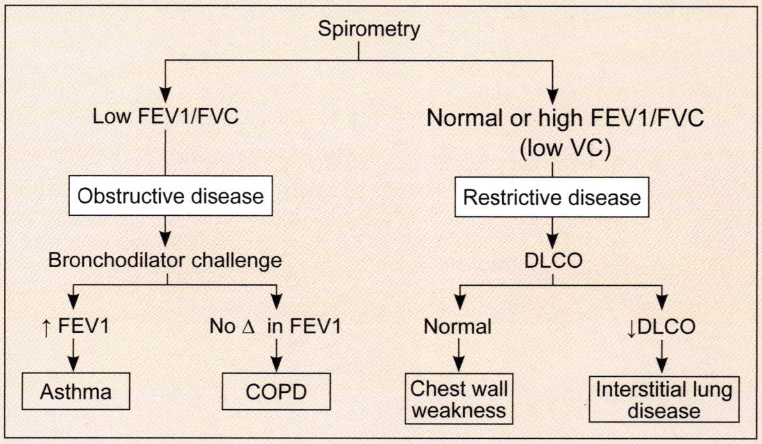

Spirometry	COPD	Restrictive lung diseases
FEV1	Low++	Low+
VC	Low+	Low++
FEV1/FVC	Low	Normal/high
RV	High	Low
FRC	High	Low

- **TLC:** Volume of air in the lungs following maximal inspiration **(N= 5-6 L)**
- **FVC:** Maximum amount of air exhaled following maximal inspiration **(N= 4.8 L)**
- **VT:** Volume of air entering and leaving lungs during normal respiration **(N= 500 ml)**
- **RV:** Volume of air remaining in the lungs after maximal expiratory effort **(N= 1.2 L)**
- **FRC:** Volume of air within the lungs at the end of normal respiration **(N= 2.5-3 L)**
- **FEV:** Volume of air exhaled in a given time during a forced vital capacity effort
- **FEV1/FVC:** Proportion of a person's vital capacity that they are able to expire in the first second of expiration **(N= 80%)**

Restrictive Lung Disease:

- **FVC is reduced** because of reduction in intra-thoracic air volume
- **Normal or Increased FEV1/FVC**
- Examples are:
  - ***Interstitial lung disease***
  - ***Neuromuscular disorders***
  - Mechanical compression like ***obesity, kyphoscoliosis, pneumothorax***
- **TLC and RV** are reduced in all except in **neuromuscular disorders.**

Obstructive Lung Disease

- Two major types:
  - COPD
  - Bronchial asthma
- Both show **reduced FEV1/FVC**
- **FEV1** is used for follow up of asthma and COPD and in evaluation of bronchodilator response
- **Reversal of obstruction** with bronchodilators **(Improvement of FEV1 >12%** and minimum **of >200 ml)** is characteristic of asthma
- A post-bronchodilator forced expiratory volume in one second (FEV1/FVC) **less than 0.7** confirms COPD.

Ans: (a) FEV1/FVC decreased

Ref: *TARGET Pediatrics (Wolters Kluwer) by Arun Babu, 1st edition, Page 378*

24. 65-year-old lady underwent mastectomy for Carcinoma breast. Later she developed frontal headache, pain in temple region and around eye. Her ESR is 55 mm/hour. What is the most probable diagnosis?

(a) Cavernous sinus thrombosis
(b) Meningeal Metastasis
(c) Frontal sinusitis
(d) Giant cell arteritis

Explanation:

GIANT CELL ARTERITIS (AKA TEMPORAL ARTERITIS)

- Inflammation of large sized arteries
- Commonly involves extracranial branches of external carotid artery
- **Most common** involved artery **– Temporal artery**
- Assciated with **polymyalgia rheumatica** (seen in 40-50% cases of GCA)
- Common in **elderly patients (> 55 years)**
- More common in **women**
- **Clinical Features**
  - Localized scalp tenderness over the temporal artery
  - Thick and nodular on palpation
  - **Jaw claudication–**Most specific symptom
  - **Visual symptoms: Diplopia** or **amaurosis fugax** (Anterior ischemic optic neuropathy)
  - Fever, Malaise, Fatigue
  - Anorexia, Loss of weight, Sweats
  - Arthralgia
- **Investigations**
  - **Elevated ESR**
  - Anemia
  - **Temporal artery biopsy–**showing giant cells – **Investigation of choice**
- **Treatment**–Oral **Prednisolone**

Ans: (d) Giant cell arteritis

Ref: *Harrison's Principles of Internal Medicine, 19th edition*

25. All except are features Plummer-Vinson syndrome:

(a) Hypertrophy of oral mucosa (b) Dysphagia

(c) Glossitis (d) Iron deficiency anemia

Explanation:

PLUMMER–VINSON SYNDROME (PVS)

- Also called **Paterson–Brown–Kelly syndrome** or **sideropenic dysphagia**
- **It is Premalignant**
- Presents as a triad of:
  - ***Dysphagia***
  - ***Esophageal webs***
  - ***Iron deficiency anemia***
- It most usually occurs in postmenopausal women.

Clinical Features

- Burning sensation with the tongue and oral mucosa
- **Atrophy of lingual papillae** produces a smooth, shiny, red dorsum of the tongue.
- Dysphagia

- Pain
- Weakness
- Odynophagia
- **Atrophic glossitis**
- Angular stomatitis
- The condition is associated with **koilonychia, glossitis, cheilitis,** and **splenomegaly**
- Hemogram – **Microcytic hypochromic** anemia suggestive of iron deficiency
- Increased risk of **squamous cell carcinoma of Esophagus**

Ans: (a) Hypertrophy of oral mucosa

Ref: *Harrison's Principles of Internal Medicine, 19th edition*

SURGERY

1. Which of the following is correct regarding treatment of Pressure sore?

(a) Surgery is the only modality of the treatment

(b) Serum albumin prior to surgical treatment is warranted

(c) Herbal remedies with or without insulin therapy is mostly useful than other remedies

(d) Stage 2 and 3 ulcers may be left to heal secondarily after debridement

Explanation:

Pressure Sore:

- **Tissue pressure > 30 mm Hg** will result in Tissue Ischemia.
- Most common site is **Ischial tuberosity*** (28%), 2nd most common site is **Greater Trochanter (19%)** and 3rd Common in **Sacrum**.
- **Muscle** is more susceptible than skin to ischemic insult due to its relatively high metabolic demand.

Stages of Pressure Sore:

- **Stage 1**, Non-blanching erythema over intact skin.
- **Stage 2**, Partial-thickness injury (epidermis or dermis)—blister or crater.
- **Stage 3,** Full-thickness injury extending down to, but not including, fascia and without undermining of adjacent tissue; and
- **Stage 4**, Full-thickness skin injury with destruction or necrosis of muscle, bone, tendon,or joint capsule.

Management:

- Management principles for pressure sores should include **pressure relief** (air mattresses and gel cushions for redistribution of pressure), **systemic optimization** (particularly nutritional support) and **wound care.**
- Goals of surgical intervention are drainage of **fluid collections**, **wide debridement** of **devitalized** and **scarred tissue**, excision of **pseudobursa**, **ostectomy** of involved **bones**, **hemostasis**, and **tension-free closure** of dead space with well-vascularized tissue (muscle, musculocutaneous, or fasciocutaneous flaps).
- **Stage 2 and 3 ulcers may be left to heal secondarily after debridement****.
- **Subatmospheric pressure wound therapy devices** (vacuum-assisted closure) play a role in wound management by removing excess interstitial fluid, promoting capillary circulation, decreasing bacterial colonization, increasing vascularity and granulation tissue formation and contributing to wound size reduction.

Ans: (d) Stage 2 and 3 ulcers may be left to heal secondarily after debridement

Ref: *Schwartz, 10th edition, Page 482*

2. Mr. Ramu, 30 years old male with Papillary carcinoma in Thyroid with a Nodule <3 cm confined to neck with 2 lymph node palpable in neck along with Lung micrometastasis. How will you stage this according to AJCC 8th Edition?

(a) I

(b) II

(c) III

(d) IV

Explanation:

AJCC 8TH EDITION: THYROID CANCER STAGING

T staging

- Tx–Primary tumor cannot be assessed
- T0–No evidence of primary tumor

T1–Tumor <2 cm in greatest dimension limited to the thyroid

- T1a – Tumor <1 cm
- T1b – Tumor 1 cm-2 cm

T2–Tumor 2-4 cm limited to the thyroid

T3–Tumor >4 cm or with extrathyroidal extension

- T3a: Tumor >4 cm in greatest dimension **limited to the thyroid.**
- T3b: Tumor of any size with **gross extrathyroidal extension** invading only strap muscles (sternohyoid, sternothyroid, thyrohyoid or omohyoid muscles).

T4: Locally Advanced

- T4a: **Moderately advanced disease**; tumor of any size with **gross extrathyroidal** extension into the nearby tissues of the neck, including subcutaneous soft tissue, larynx, trachea, esophagus, or recurrent laryngeal nerve.
- T4b: **Very advanced disease**; tumor of any size with extension toward the spine or into nearby large blood vessels, invading the prevertebral fascia, or encasing the carotid artery or mediastinal vessels.

All T categories must be subdivided into Solitary (S) or Multifocal (M), in Multifocal-Largest dimension taken for T staging.

N staging:

N0–No evidence of locoregional lymph node

- N0a: One or more cytologically or histologically confirmed benign lymph nodes
- N0b: No radiologic or clinical evidence of locoregional lymph node metastasis

N1- Metastasis to regional nodes

- N1a: Metastasis to level VI or VII lymph nodes
- N1b: Unilateral, Bilateral or contralateral cervical (Levels I - V) or retropharyngeal or superior mediastinal lymph nodes (Level VII).

M1–Metastasis

Changes made by 8th Edition:

- T3 is subdivided into T3a and T3b by 8th Edition.
- AJCC Stage Grouping from AJCC manual, please note the interesting point in this, the stage grouping is based on Age.
- Age < 55 years having only Stage I and Stage II and no other stages.
- Stage I is with no mets and Stage II is with mets.
- Naturally most of you would have put Stage IV and that's wrong at this age given in the question.

When age at diagnosis is...	And T is...	And N is...	And M is...	Then the stage group is...
< 55 years	Any T	Any N	M0	I
< 55 years	Any T	Any N	M1	II
≥ 55 years	T1	N0/NX	M0	I
≥ 55 years	T1	N1	M0	II
≥ 55 years	T2	N0/NX	M0	I
≥ 55 years	T2	N1	M0	II
≥ 55 years	T3a/T3b	Any N	M0	II
≥ 55 years	T4a	Any N	M0	III
≥ 55 years	T4b	Any N	M0	IVA
≥ 55 years	Any	Any N	M1	IVB

Ans: (b) Stage II

Ref: *AJCC, 8th edition, Page 883*

3. Most common site of Curling ulcer is:

(a) Stomach
(b) 1st part of duodenum
(c) 2nd part of duodenum
(d) Junction between 2nd and 3rd part of duodenum

Explanation:

- **Curling's ulcer** is an acute gastric erosion resulting as a complication from **severe burns** when reduced plasma volume leads to ischemia and cell necrosis (sloughing) of the gastric mucosa.
- In a study among burns patients, 135 patients (mean age, 49.5±13.5 years) underwent endoscopy.
- Endoscopy revealed ulcer in 51 patients:
  - **36 (70.6%) with gastric ulcers (Most common now)**
  - 9 (17.6%) with duodenal ulcers
  - 6 (11.8%) with both
- In this study, the rate of ulcer was higher in patient who had a burn area >20% of TBSA compared with patients with a burn area <20% of TBSA.

Ans: (a) Stomach

Ref: *Based on a Journal in 2015–Revised risk analysis of stress ulcers in burn patients receiving ulcer prophylaxis, Young Hwan Choi*

4. Hernia not related to abdominal wall:

(a) Amyand hernia
(b) Richter hernia
(c) Littre hernia
(d) Peterson hernia

Explanation:

- **Petersen hernias** are internal hernias which occur in the potential space posterior to a **gastrojejunostomy**. This hernia is caused by the herniation of intestinal loops through the defect between the small bowel limbs, the transverse mesocolon and the retroperitoneum, after any type of gastrojejunostomy.

Various Types of Hernias

- **Spigelian hernia**–Via the Arcuate line infra umbilical.
- **Richter's hernia**–A part of circumference is obstructed (Diarrhea+).
- **Peterson Hernia**–Hernia behind Roux Limb.
- **Stammers Hernia**–Hernia behind Transverse mesocolon.
- **Ogilvie's Hernia**–Via a defect in Conjoint Tendon.

- **Laugier's Hernia**–Via defect in Lacunar ligament.
- **Littre Hernia**–Meckel's diverticulum containing hernia.
- **Amyand Hernia**–Appendix containing hernia.
- **Berger's Hernia**–Hernia into Pouch of Doughals.
- **Grynfelt Hernia**–Superior lumbar hernia.
- **Petit Hernia**–Inferior lumbar hernia.
- **Narath Hernia**–Hernia seen in congenital Dislocation of hip.
- **Maydl's Hernia**–W' shaped loop in hernial sac. Retrograde strangulation occurs.
- **Cloquet's Hernia** is one in which the sac lies under the fascia covering the pectineus muscle.
- **Gibbon's Hernia**–Hernia with hydrocele.
- **Beclard's Hernia**–Femoral hernia via opening in Saphenous Vein**.

Ans: (d) Peterson hernia

Ref: *Surgery Sixer, 4th edition, Page 507*

5. Which is not true regarding breast cancer in pregnancy?

(a) Mammography is a diagnostic modality in breast cancer
(b) Behaves in a similar way to breast cancer in a non-pregnant young woman
(c) Most tumors are hormone receptor negative
(d) Ductal carcinoma is most common type

Explanation:

BREAST CANCER DURING PREGNANCY

- 1 in 3000 pregnancy.
- **Axillary nodes** are positive in 75%.
- Average age= **34 years.**
- **Mammography** is **NOT** indicated in pregnancy and advice only **USG and Needle Biopsy**.
- **Ductal carcinoma*** is most common type.
- Most tumors are hormone receptor **negative.**
- Because of the potential deleterious effects of radiation therapy on the fetus, **radiation cannot be considered until the fetus is delivered.**
- A **modified radical mastectomy*** can be performed during the **first* and second* trimesters** of pregnancy.
- **During the third trimester, lumpectomy*** with axillary node dissection can be considered if adjuvant radiation therapy is deferred until after delivery.
- **Lactation is suppressed**.
- **Chemotherapy administered during the first trimester carries a risk of spontaneous abortion and a 12% risk of birth defects.** There is no evidence of teratogenicity resulting from administration of chemotherapeutic agents in the second and third trimesters.
- For this reason, many clinicians now consider the optimal strategy to be delivery of chemotherapy in the **second and third trimesters as a neoadjuvant approach**, which allows local therapy decisions to be made after the delivery of the baby.
- Pregnant women with breast cancer often present at a **later stage** of disease because breast tissue changes that occur in the hormone-rich environment of pregnancy obscure early cancers.
- **However, pregnant women with breast cancer have a prognosis, stage by stage, that is similar to that of nonpregnant women with breast cancer**.**

Ans: (a) Mammography is a diagnostic modality in breast cancer

Ref: *Schwartz, 10th edition, Page 554*

6. A patient underwent complicated surgery for chronic pancreatitis. The most preferred route for supplementary nutrition in this patient would be:

(a) Total parenteral nutrition
(b) Feeding gastrostomy
(c) Feeding jejunostomy
(d) Oral feeding

Explanation:

Procedures done for Chronic Pancreatitis

Drainage Procedures	Resection+ Drainage Procedures
1. For dilated duct: > 7 mm diameter: - Modified Puestow procedure **2. For Undilated duct:** - Izbicki Procedure in which V' Shaped excision of the duct done.	**With head mass:** **1. Whipple's procedure (not done nowadays)** **2. Duodenum Preserving Pancreatic head resection (DPPHR)** - Beger's Procedure - Bern's Modification - Frey's Procedure

- The resection with drainage procedures are all complicated surgeries and the nutrition will be started by a Feeding Jejunostomy Tube which will be inserted during the surgery.
- The purpose of Feeding Jejunostomy is, even if there is a leak from Pancreatic Jejunostomy anastomosis we can feed the patient as we have kept the tube distal to the anastomosis.

Ans: (c) Feeding jejunostomy

Ref: *Practical Question (Based on Surgery Sixer, 4th edition)*

7. A 25-year-old college student met with road traffic accident and is admitted in casualty. He has marked abdominal distension, pulse rate of 140 and a BP of 80/50 mm Hg. The most appropriate initial investigation would be:

(a) Abdominal paracentesis
(b) CT abdomen
(c) Plain X-ray of abdomen
(d) FAST scan

Explanation:

The Blunt Trauma Abdomen Protocol is a frequent question–please read it

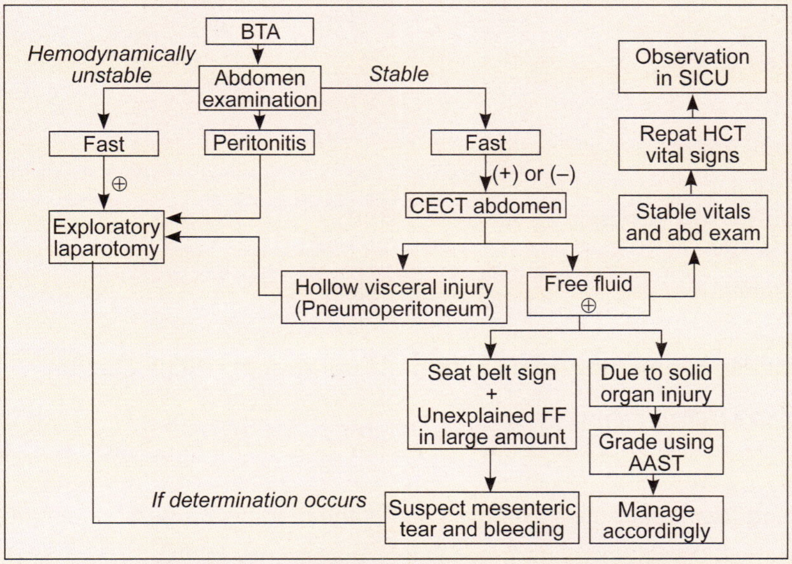

Flowchart: Management of blunt trauma abdomen (BTA)

Ans: (d) FAST scan

Ref: *Surgery Sixer, 4th edition, Page 94*

8. A 50-year-old lady with history of carcinoid syndrome complains of flushing and diarrhea. Which of the following is not true regarding this syndrome?

(a) Occurs in <10% of carcinoid tumors
(b) Octreotide injection reduces symptoms of flushing and diarrhea
(c) Attacks precipitated by stress, alcohol and large meal
(d) Bright-red patchy flushing is typically seen with Ileal carcinoids

Explanation:

- **Malignant carcinoid syndrome** develops only if **liver metastases** develop; because all the hormones are detoxified in liver. The only exceptions to get **Carcinoid syndrome** in **absence** of **Liver mets** are – **Ovarian** and **Retroperitoneal carcinoids** as their drainage is directly systemic and not portal.

Carcinoid syndrome:

- Vasomotor symptoms (80%: Cutaneous flushing is the most common symptom**.
- GIT: Explosive diarrhea. Due to serotonin.
- **Cardiovascular:** The three most common cardiac lesions are pulmonary stenosis (90%), tricuspid insufficiency (47%), and tricuspid stenosis (42%)***.
- **Asthmatic attacks:** Bronchospasm.
- Malabsorption and pellagra (dementia, diarrhea, dermatitis) due to excessive diversion of tryptophan.
- **Types of flushing:** Diffuse erythematous, violaceous, prolonged flushes and bright red patchy.
- Most common type of flushing seen in **gastric carcinoids**: **Bright red patchy**. (**Not** in **Ileal Carcinoids**).
- **Octreotide** reduces these symptoms.
- **Stress** and a **Huge meal** increases these symptoms.

Ans: (d) Bright red patchy flushing is typically seen in ileal carcinoids

Ref: *Surgery Sixer, 4th edition, Page 411*

9. A patient with necrotising fasciitis is treated with antibiotics and debridement. He got discharged on wound recovery. Now he came back after 10 days with diarrhea and fever. The following are done except:

(a) Continue same antibiotic
(b) Stop Loperamide 2 mg
(c) Metronidazole is the Drug of Choice
(d) Washing hands with alcohol based hand sanitizers are superior to washing hands with soap to stop the spread of diarrhea

Explanation:

This is a case of **Pseudomembranous colitis (Clostridium Difficile Colitis)**

PSEUDOMEMBRANOUS COLITIS

Introduction:

- ***C. difficile colitis*** is extremely common and is the leading cause of nosocomially acquired diarrhea.
- The spectrum of disease ranges from watery diarrhea to fulminant, life-threatening colitis. *C. difficile* is carried in the large intestine of many healthy adults.

- Colitis is thought to result from overgrowth of this organism after depletion of the normal commensal flora of the gut with the use of antibiotics.
- Although **clindamycin** was the first antimicrobial agent associated with *C. difficile* colitis, almost any antibiotic may cause this disease.

Predisposing Factors:

- Moreover, although the risk of *C. difficile* colitis increases with prolonged antibiotic use, even a single dose of an antibiotic may cause the disease.
- Immunosuppression, medical comorbidities, prolonged hospitalization or nursing home residence, and bowel surgery increase the risk.

Diagnosis:

- Diagnosis of this disease was traditionally made by **culturing the organism from the stool**.
- **Detection** of **one or both toxins** (either by cytotoxic assays or by immunoassays) has proven to be more rapid, sensitive and specific.
- The diagnosis may also be made endoscopically by detection of characteristic ulcers, plaques and pseudo membranes.

Management:

- **Immediate cessation*** of the offending antimicrobial agent.
- Mild disease treated as outpatients with a **10-day course of oral metronidazole**.
- **Oral vancomycin** is a second-line agent used in patients allergic to metronidazole or in patients with recurrent disease.
- **Loperamide** and other motility agents are **contraindicated** as they stagnate the toxin in Lumen and cause more symptoms.
- Reintroduction of normal floraby ingestion of ***probiotics* or *stool transplantation*** has been suggested as a possible treatment for recurrent or refractory disease.
- **Fulminant colitis***, characterized by septicemia and/or evidence of perforation, requires emergent laparotomy. A total **abdominal colectomy with end ileostomy** may be lifesaving.

Ans: (a) Continue same antibiotic

Ref: *Schwartz, 10th edition, Page 1222; Studies from Internet Sources*

10. Shrugging of shoulder following neck surgery due to injury to:

(a) Spinal Accessory Nerve
(b) Thoracodorsal Nerve
(c) Bell's Nerve
(d) Vagus Nerve

Explanation:

Radical Neck Node Dissection of CRILE'S:

- The classic operation involves **resection** of the **cervical lymphatics** and **lymph nodes** and those structures closely associated:
  - **The internal jugular vein**
  - **The accessory nerve**
  - **The sternocleidomastoid muscle**
- These structures are all removed *en bloc* and in continuity with the primary disease if possible.
- The main disability that follows the operation is **weakness** and **drooping of the shoulder** due to paralysis of the **trapezius** muscle as a consequence of excision of the **accessory nerve***.

Ans: (a) Spinal Accessory Nerve

Ref: *Bailey and Love, 27th edition, Page 758*

11. Image of X-ray with superior mediastinal mass. Probable diagnosis:

(a) Thymoma
(b) Prevertebral abscess
(c) Lymphoma
(d) Aortic aneurysm

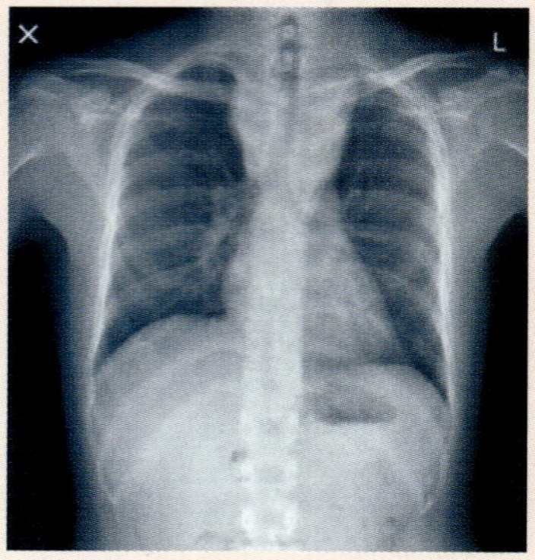

Explanation:

- Bailey explains with an illustrated picture of the various mediastinal masses.
- The picture shows clearly a Superior Mediastinal mass.
- The various superior mediastinal masses are:
  - **Lymphoma**
  - **Thyroid Extension**
  - **Parathyroid**

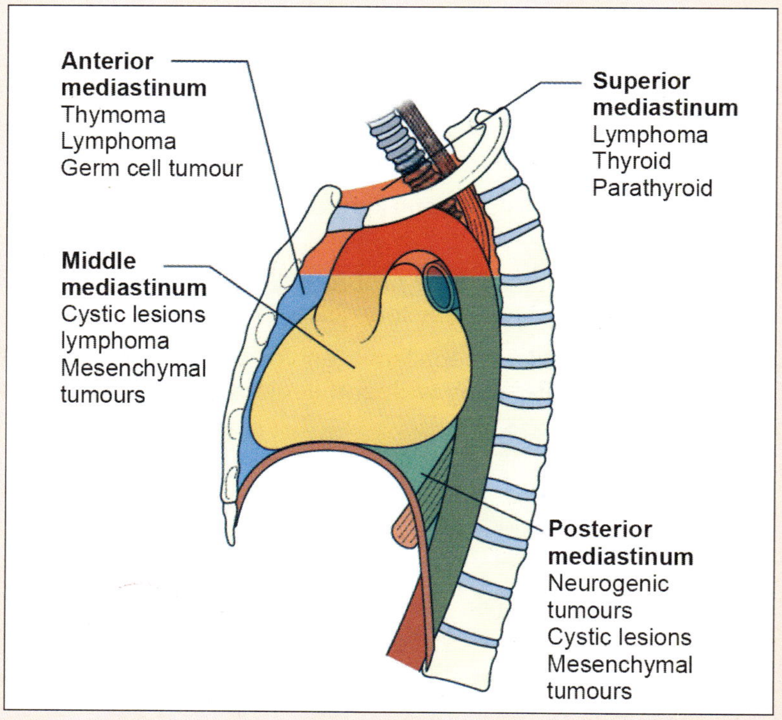

Ans: (c) Lymphoma

Ref: *Bailey and Love, 27th edition, Page 935*

12. All are true regarding Inferior pedicle breast surgery except:

(a) It is a technique used for Reduction Mammoplasty
(b) This procedure is contraindicated in smoking females
(c) Lactation is possible always after the surgery
(d) The removed breast tissue is sent for pathological study always

Explanation:

Reduction Mammaplasty:

- The principles guiding reduction mammaplasty for breast hypertrophy are:
  - To improve the patient's symptoms
  - To decrease the volume of the breast
  - To reshape the breast to correct ptosis
  - To elevate the breast tissue to an anatomically correct position on the chest wall
  - To reposition the nipple and areola on the reduced and reshaped breast
  - To preserve the nerve supply to the skin and nipple-areola complex
  - To maintain blood supply to the breast tissue, and
  - To minimize scars.
- Surgical techniques are described by the location of the block of tissue to which the nipple and areola are left attached and by the pattern of incisions and subsequent scars.
  - **Inferior pedicle technique is used most commonly**
  - Other techniques are central, superior, medial, lateral, and doubly attached vertical and horizontal pedicles. All variants are designed to maximize blood supply while allowing adequate tissue removal.
- All variants are designed to maximize blood supply while allowing adequate tissue removal.

Prerequisites for Reduction mammaplasty:

- All patients >35 years must undergo mammography to rule out cancer.
- The removed breast tissue must be sent for HPE.
- No set lower age limit for this surgery.
- In adolescents we must do reduction only when the breast stops growing for at least 12 months.
- 2nd Time Breast Reduction is not done due to risk of loss of blood supply to breast.
- Post Radiation to Breast patients are delayed for surgery.
- Smoking is a contraindication for Breast Reduction.
- Obese patients has high complication rates.

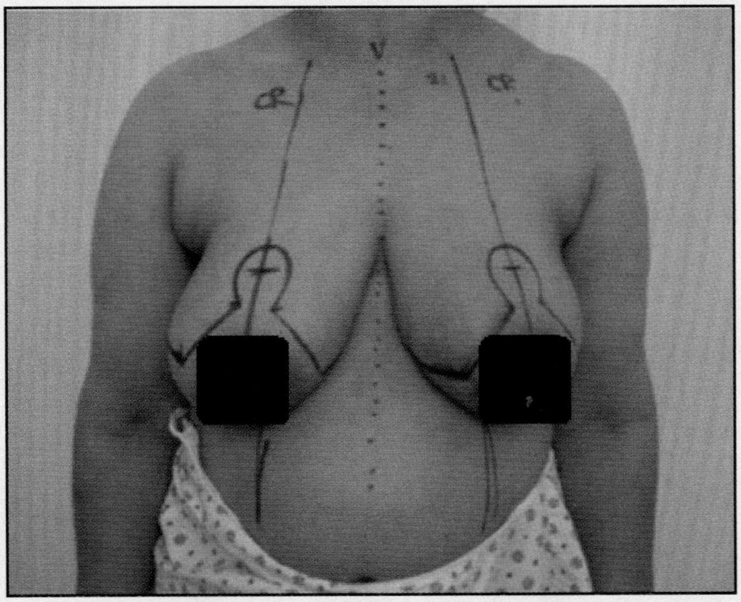

Figure: Inferior pedicle technique of reduction mammaplasty

Complications of Breast Reduction Techniques:

- Lactation and **breastfeeding** are not possible.
- Changes in **Nipple sensation** (More of increased sensation than decreased sensation).
- Wound **dehiscence**, skin slough, loss of tissue, hematoma, infection, and fat necrosis.

Ans: (c) Lactation is possible always after the surgery

Ref: *Sabiston, 20th edition, Page 1955*

13. Which are the following is not true regarding Charcot-Bouchard aneurysm?

(a) Causes Spontaneous Intracerebral Hemorrhage

(b) They are micro aneurysms

(c) Most commonly located in anterior cerebral artery

(d) Hemorrhage is most common in putamen

Explanation:

Spontaneous Intracerebral Hemorrhages:

- Spontaneous intracerebral hemorrhages into the brain parenchyma are common, accounting for approximately 10% of all strokes.
- They generally occur in older patients, usually because of degenerative changes in the cerebral vessels that are often associated with **chronic hypertension**.
- In younger patients, they are more likely related to **drug abuse or vascular malformation**.
- They can occur anywhere in the cerebral circulation or brainstem but are classically described in association with ***small degenerative aneurysms (microaneurysms; also known as Charcot-Bouchard aneurysms)*** at the junctions of the perforating vessels and larger vessels at the skull base.
- They are typically on the **middle cerebral artery junctions** with the small perforating lenticulostriate vessels, **leading to hemorrhage into the putamen**.

Clinical Features:

- Stroke features.
- Symptoms are more likely to include headache than ischemic stroke.

Diagnosis:

- The diagnosis is with CT, usually done in an emergency department setting.
- Further investigation is generally done with contrast MRI or magnetic resonance angiography. Any suggestion of aneurysm or AVM is followed by conventional catheter angiography.

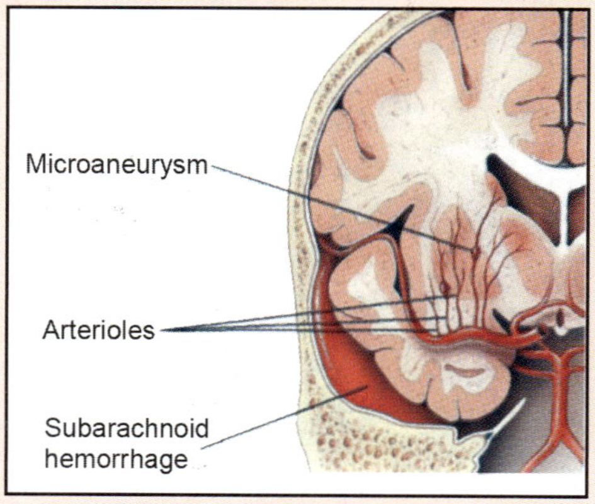

Figure: Showing Charcot-Bouchard aneurysms in middle cerebral artery

Ans: (c) Most commonly located in anterior cerebral artery

Ref: *Sabiston 20th edition, Page 1906*

14. 40-year-old male patient with tumor size 5 cm with no mediastinal node was diagnosed with Small cell cancer lung with no metastasis. What is the correct treatment for this condition?

(a) Only Chemotherapy
(b) Surgical resection with Chemotherapy
(c) Radiotherapy + Chemotherapy
(d) Only Surgical resection

Explanation:

Primary Lung cancer (From Bailey and Love 27th Edition)

- Most common cause of cancer death in the world.
- Most common cancer in the world.
- Most common risk factor is smoking.

Histological Subtypes:

Small Cell Lung Cancer	Non Small Cell Lung Cancers
• A type of NET • 20% of all Lung cancers • Extensive Early Lymph node and hematogenous mets seen • Worst prognosis of < 5% survival at 5 years • This is the tumor responsive to Chemotherapy at the best in spite of being bad prognosis the survival is increased few months with Chemotherapy	• Adeno cancer is the most common now and has overtaken the SCC • Squamous cell cancer is a cavitating cancer • Large cell is a type of NET • Bronchioalveolar carcinoma (old name–Adenocarcinoma in situ)–New Name–"***Lepidic Neoplastic lesions***" o Ground glass appearance o Multifocal Primary Tumors+

Essential Clinical Features:

- Most common symptom is Hemoptysis (<50% cases).
- Ominous feature–Pleural fluid with blood.
- Small cell cancer has Eaton Myasthenic Lambert Syndrome**.
- Pancoast Tumor is a feature of Squamous type–Causes Horner's Syndrome.
- SVC syndrome is a feature of small cell cancer.

TNM staging of Lung Cancer (Simplified version)

T Staging
- T1–< 3 cm
- T2–3-5 cm or Involves main Bronchus, Involves Visceral Pleura or Having Lung Atelectasis.
- T3–5-7 cm or Involves Chest wall, parietal pleura, Phrenic nerve, Parietal pericardium and Superior Sulcus. Tumors.
- T4–> 7 cm lesion or Involves Diaphragm, Heart, great vessels, Esophagus, Vertebra, Carina, Recurrent Laryngeal nerve.

N Staging
- N1–Ipsilateral Peribronchial and Hilar nodes.
- N2–Ipsilateral Mediastinal and Subcarinal nodes.
- N3–Contralateral any node.

M Staging
- M1a–Tumor with Contralateral lobe nodules, Pleural or Pericardial Nodules.
- M1b–Single Extra Thoracic Mets.
- M1c–Multiple Extra Thoracic Mets in one or more organs.

Investigations:

- X-ray Chest diagnoses most cancer.
- 1st Investigation in Suspected Lung Cancer–**CECT Thorax** (>2 cm nodes are mostly metastatic).
- IOC to look for mets–**PET CT***.
- Sputum cytology–May reveal malignant cells but False negative rate is high.

Biopsy Procedures:

- Centrally Located tumors–Bronchoscopy and Transbronchial Needle Aspiration (**TBNA**).
- Peripherally Located tumors–Percutaneous CT guided Biopsy.

Surgical Staging:

- In cases of Doubtful involvement of Nodes direct nodal biopsy done by three methods.
- Mediastinoscopy via a 2 cm incision above suprasternal notch.
- Mediastinotomy via an incision in 2nd ICS on affected side.
- VATS Biopsy of Nodes.

Surgical Treatment:

- Thoracotomy – Most frequent indication of Thoracotomy is **Lung cancer**.
- Double lumen Endotracheal tube inserted and operative side lung collapsed.
- Patient put in left lateral position with affected lung up.
- Incision made below scapula tip.
- Nowadays Lung cancer surgery done by VATS.

- Surgery with Curative intent is possible upto T1-T3 tumors and N0-N1 cases only.
- For Non Small Cell Lung cancer surgery is done with CURATIVE INTENT, even T3 tumors involving chest wall is resected enbloc.

Types of Surgery for Lung Cancer:

Segmentectomy and Wedge Resection	Lobectomy	Pneumonectomy	Bronchoplastic Lung Resection
• For Small tumors. • Ligate the segmental Pulmonary artery and vein and Bronchus.	• **Early stage Lung cancer** this is the **Treatment of Choice**. • The Pulmonary artery and vein with bronchus supplying the lobe is ligated. • 2-3% mortality.	• Removal of whole lung. • Indicated for Centrally located Tumors or those tumors crossing the main fissures. • Main Pulmonary artery and Superior and inferior Pulmonary vein ligated. Main bronchus is divided. • Drainage of the space is done without suction. Air in the space is gradually replaced by fluid level.	• To avoid complications related to lung resection, lung tissue preservative operation is done. • Sleeve lung resection of centrally located tumor with reanastomosis of Cut major Bronchus to remaining lobar bronchus.

Complications of Lung Resection:

- Bleeding
- Respiratory Infection
- Persistent Air leak
- Broncho pleural fistula–Most serious Complication. Higher Morbidity and Mortality seen.

PROGNOSIS OF LUNG CANCERS:

Five-year Survival Rate

- Squamous cell cancer–35-50%
- Adenocarcinoma–25-45%
- Small cell cancer–0-5%

Ans: (b) Surgical resection with chemotherapy

Ref: *Bailey and Love, 27th edition, Page 928-931*

15. Desmoid Tumor is associated with:

(a) Colonic polyps (b) Pancreatic cancer
(c) Ovarian cancer (d) Gastric cancer

Explanation:

*"Desmoid tumours are commonly associated with **familial adenomatous polyposis (FAP)**, in which **colonic polyps** are the most common feature".*

DESMOID TUMOUR

- Desmoid tumor, also known as **fibromatosis or aggressive fibromatosis**.
- It is an uncommon neoplasm that occurs sporadically or as part of an inherited syndrome associated with:
  - **Familial adenomatous polyposis (FAP).**
  - **Gardner's syndrome**, an autosomal dominant syndrome of ***GI adenomatous polyps*** or ***adenocarcinoma***, ***osteomas*** and ***skin and soft tissue tumors***.

Pathophysiology

- Arise from fibroaponeurotic tissue; and
- Lack metastatic potential.
- Locally aggressive and invasive, with a high propensity for recurrence.
- Associated with Oral contraceptive use.
- Estrogen receptors are present within the tumor; suggest a regulatory role for estrogen in this disease.

Classification

Desmoid tumors are typically classified by location:

- ***Extra-abdominal or extremity desmoids*** (i.e., those tumors occurring in the proximal extremities or limb girdle).
- ***Abdominal wall tumors.***
- ***Intra-abdominal desmoids***, which involve the mesentery, pelvis, or bowel wall.

Clinical Features

- Majority of desmoid tumors are **sporadic**.
- Typically in **young women** during **pregnancy** or **within a year of childbirth**.
- Typically present as a **slowly growing** mass.
- Usually present with an asymptomatic mass or with symptoms related to mass effect from the tumor.
- Often a temporal association between the discovery of the tumor and an antecedent history of abdominal trauma or operation.

Investigations

- ***Imaging (CT or MRI)*** is necessary to delineate the extent of tumor involvement fully.
- No need to perform staging for metastatic disease.
- ***Biopsy*** is required to establish the diagnosis.
- ***Core needle biopsy or incisional biopsy*** will demonstrate a tumor composed of bundles of spindle cells and an abundant fibrous stroma.
- **Immunohistochemistry** can help clarify difficult diagnoses.
- Typically stain **positive for β-catenin, actin and vimentin** and **stain negative for cytokeratin and S-100.**

MANAGEMENT

Surgery

- **Surgery** is the treatment of choice.
- Resection of the tumor with a wide margin of normal tissue is the optimal treatment.
- Often, the extent of this resection will require abdominal wall reconstruction with local tissue flaps or mesh prostheses.

Radiation

- Abdominal wall desmoids are responsive to radiation therapy, although the treatment effect is slow and may be progressive over several years.

Radiotherapy as Primary Treatment

- Radiotherapy alone is an acceptable treatment option for patients with ***unresectable desmoid tumors*** or tumors for which resection will be associated with high morbidity risks or major functional loss.

Adjuvant Radiotherapy

- Adjuvant radiation therapy is **controversial**, with most centers reserving this modality for **patients with positive margins, or close margins**

Neoadjuvant Radiotherapy

- The use of neo-adjuvant radiation therapy is **less well accepted** than adjuvant radiation therapy because of the slow response times, **often 1 year or more**, with the potential for making subsequent abdominal wall reconstruction more difficult, and few studies demonstrating a clear benefit.

Adjuvant Medical Therapy

- ***Tamoxifen.***
- NSAIDS particularly Indomethacin and Sulindac.
- ***Imatinib***–A tyrosine kinase inhibitor.
- ***Chemotherapy***–Methotrexate with vinblastine, doxorubicin-based therapy, and ifosfamide-based regimens.
- For **desmoids with rapid growth**, medical oncologists may recommend therapies typically used for sarcomas, such as **doxorubicin and dacarbazine.**

Ans: (a) Colonic polyps

Ref: *Sabiston Textbook of Surgery, 19th edition, Page 1095*

16. Most common presentation of Retroperitoneal fibrosis is:

(a) Bilateral pedal edema (b) Ascites

(c) Ureteral obstruction (d) Back pain

Explanation:

*"The first complaint is invariably **dull**, **noncolicky** pain. It usually originates in the flank or **low back** and often radiates to the **lower abdomen**, **groin**, **genitalia**, or **anteromedial aspect** of the **thigh**." Ref: Schwartz*

*"Most patients present with **ureteric obstruction**, often with **renal failure.**" Ref: Bailey*

*"The most common symptom (**92%** of cases) is a dull, **poorly localized**, **noncolicky pain** in the **flank**, back, scrotum, or lower abdomen." Ref: Medscape*

Idiopathic Retroperitoneal Fibrosis

- **Path:** Extensive collagen deposition surrounds the ureters, mostly at the level of the pelvic brim or below. Most patients present with ***ureteric obstruction***, often with ***renal failure.***
- Cases due to malignancy are treated appropriately according to the cause.
- This is a ***nonspecific***, ***nonsuppurative*** inflammation of ***fibroadipose*** tissue that produces symptoms by the ***gradual compression*** of the ***tubular structures*** in the retroperitoneal space.
- Considered as one of the components of a widespread disease, ***Systemic idiopathic fibrosis.***
- Other components of Systemic idiopathic fibrosis are:
  - Idiopathic mediastinal fibrosis
  - Riedel's struma
  - Sclerosing cholangitis
  - Panniculitis
  - Peyronie's disease
  - Desmoid tumor
- The lesion consists of a plaque of woody, white fibrous tissue that is distributed along the course of the periaortic lymphatics.
- In about ***one-third*** of patients it is ***bilateral***.
- The involved tissue surrounds and constricts but does not invade the regional structures in the retroperitoneum.
- The pattern varies from a subacute cellular process with polymorphonuclear cells, lymphocytes, fibroblasts, and fat cells to a completely hyalinized, relatively acellular sclerosis.

Clinical Manifestations

- 2-3 times more common in men.
- Two-thirds of patients are 40–60 years old.
- The first complaint is often ***dull, noncolicky pain*** in the ***flank or low back*** and often radiates to the lower abdomen, groin, genitalia, or anteromedial aspect of the thigh.
- The pain is ***unilateral*** at first but may become bilateral later, as the fibrotic process spreads.
- Moderate fever and leukocytosis present.
- Raised ESR.
- A ***transabdominal or pelvic mass*** is palpable in about one-third of patients.
- Symptoms due to ***compression of the tubular retroperitoneal structures*** may follow the initial complaints by ***1 month to 2 years***.
- The major structures involved are the:
  - Ureters
  - Aorta
  - Inferior vena cava

- ***Ureteral obstruction*** occurs in **75–85** cases.
- ***Oliguria or anuria with uremia*** in **40%** cases.
- ***Lower extremity edema*** occasionally.
- ***Arterial insufficiency*** due to fibrous constriction of the aorta or iliac arteries is uncommon.

Investigations

- **CT scan** shows a homogeneous, soft tissue mass enveloping the ureters, aorta and inferior vena cava. **Pyelogram:** A ***triad*** that is highly suggestive of retroperitoneal fibrosis.
    - Hydronephrosis with a dilated, tortuous upper ureter.
    - Medial deviation of the ureter.
    - Extrinsic ureteral compression.

Treatment

- ***Indications for surgery***
    - Onset of urinary infection.
    - Depression of renal function.
- **Steroid**-induced regression of the inflammatory edema may reestablish urinary patency – Temporary relief of symptoms.
- ***Ureterolysis with intraperitoneal transplantation*** is currently the most effective means of relieving obstruction of the involved ureter.
- ***Aortic or iliac artery obstruction*** is best treated by **arteriolysis** or **bypass** with a synthetic vascular graft.
- Symptoms due to ***venous obstruction*** are best treated with **elevation and elastic support** to the lower limbs until a sufficient collateral venous system develops.

Ans: (d) Back pain

Ref: *Bailey and Love's Short Practice of Surgery, 25th edition and Schwartz's Principles of Surgery, 9th edition and Medscape online*

OBSTETRICS AND GYNECOLOGY

1. True statement regarding Renal changes in Preeclampsia:

(a) Increased GFR
(b) Glomeruloendotheliosis
(c) Increased renal blood flow
(d) Persistent after delivery

Explanation

Renal Changes in Preeclampsia:

- Enlarged glomerulus-**glomeruloendotheliosis***
- Interstitial cells proliferate
- Spasm of afferent arterioles
- **Reduced GFR***
- Reduced tubular absorption
- Recovery complete after delivery
- **Bilateral renal cortical necrosis*** occur in severe cases

Specific organ damage in preeclampsia	
Organ	**Damage caused due to preeclampsia**
Blood vessels	Vasospasm
Kidney	Glomerular endotheliosis
Liver	Periportal hemorrhagic necrosis, subcapsular hemorrhage
Lungs	Pulmonary edema
Heart	Subendothelial hemorrhages focal necrosis
Brain	Cerebral hemorrhage, edema
Hematology	Hemoconcentration, thrombocytopenia, disseminated intravascular coagulation

Ans: (b) Glomeruloendotheliosis

Ref: *Clinical Obstetrics and Gynecology by Sharmila Arun Babu, Wolters Kluwer, 1st edition, Page 78*

2. During delivery, the baby's head was delivered but shoulders not delivered after one minute. What's the next step?

(a) Emergency LSCS
(b) Cleidotomy
(c) Lateral traction
(d) Mc Roberts maneuver

Explanation:

Shoulder Dystocia

- Occurs when anterior or posterior shoulder impacts on the maternal symphysis or on sacral promontory
- **Incidence** 0.2 to 1%
- **Causes**–Macrosomia, diabetes, obesity, postmaturity, multiparity, anencephaly, fetal ascites
- **Complications**–Fetal asphyxia, Erb's palsy, Klumpke's palsy, humerus fracture, clavicle fracture, sternomastoid hematoma, cervical and vaginal laceration, perineal tear, rupture uterus

- **Diagnosis – turtle neck sign–**recoil of the head back against the perineum, face becomes plethoric
- **Management**
  - Call for help
  - Don't give traction on head
  - Don't apply fundal pressure
  - Involve the anesthetist and pediatrician
  - Suprapubic pressure towards the chest side of the baby which will disimpact the shoulder
  - **Mc Roberts maneuver–**abduct the maternal thighs and hyperflex on to the abdomen
  - **Wood's maneuver–**posterior shoulder is rotated to anterior by cork screw movement by inserting 2 fingers in the posterior vagina
  - **"All Fours" position–**changing the position to "all Fours" position will free the impacted shoulder
  - **Cleidotomy–**deliberate fracture of the clavicle by finger pressure in an anencephalic baby or a dead fetus
  - **Zavanelli maneuver–**pushing the fetus back to the uterus and delivering by caesarean section
  - **Symphysiotomy–**done rarely

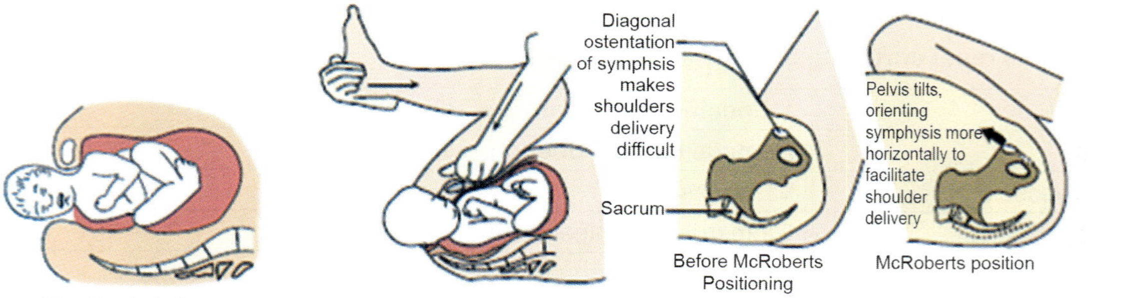

Shoulder dystocia

a. b.

McRoberts maneuver. a. Mother's legs are hyperflexed onto the abdomen along with suprapubic pressure b. The sacrum straightens and the pubic symphysis tilts anteriorly, reducing the angle of inclination

Ans: (d) Mc Roberts maneuver

Ref : *Clinical Obstetrics and Gynecology by Sharmila Arun Babu, Wolters Kluwer, 1st edition, Page 73*

3. A 30 years female is on warfarin for Deep vein thrombosis. Which contraceptive should not be advised?

(a) Progesterone only pills (b) Levonorgestrel
(c) IUCD (d) Implanon

Explanation:

Implanon

- **Progesterone** only delivery system containing **68 mg of etonogestrel**
- It releases **60 mcg** per day **over 3 years**
- It **inhibits ovulation** and causes **atrophy of the endometrium**
- It is inserted **subdermally 6-8 cm** above the **elbow fold**
- **Contraindications:**
  - Breast cancer
  - Diabetes

- Migraine
- Coronary artery disease
- Stroke
- Deep vein thrombosis
- Arterial thrombosis
- Liver failure

Contraceptive subdermal implants: Features, dosage and duration of action		
Norplant 1	**Norplant 2**	**Implanon**
6 Silastic rods	2 Silastic rods	Single polymer rod
34 mm long, 2.4 mm wide	43 mm long, 2.5 mm wide	40 mm long, 2 mm wide
Levonorgestrel 36 mg each	Levonorgestrel 70 mg each	Etonogestrel 68 mg each
Releases 85 μg/day for 6 months, 50 μg/day for 15 months, 30 μg/day thereafter	Releases 50 μg/day	Release 30 μg/day
Effective for 5 years	Effective for 3-5 years	Effective for 3 years

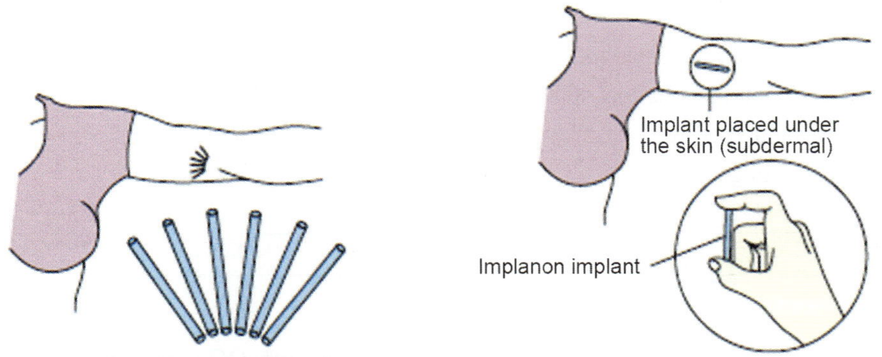

Norplant subdemal implant. Six rods are implanted in the upper inner arm

Implanon implant. One rod is placed subdermally in the upper inner arm

Ans: (d) Implanon

Ref: *DC Dutta Textbook of Obstetrics, Page 509*

4. All of the following are normal in pregnancy except:

(a) ALT and AST
(b) Prothrombin time
(c) ALP
(d) GGT

Explanation:

- With the exception of **raised ALP level**, other liver function tests like S.bilirubin, AST, ALT, CPK, LDH are unchanged in pregnancy.

Changes in liver function during pregnancy
• Fall in o Serum total protein o Serum albumin • Increase in o Binding proteins o Fibrinogen

Contd.

Contd.

o Transferrin o Ceruloplasmin o Alkaline phosphatase • Increase in portal venous pressure

Changes in gastrointestinal system during pregnancy
• Anatomical changes o Upward displacement of stomach and intestines o Gum hypertrophy o Change in the position of appendix • Physiological changes o Due to smooth muscle relaxation by – Progesterone – Estrogen-mediated released of NO o Decrease in gastric tone and motility o Increase in gastroesophageal reflux – Gastric compression by gravid uterus – Relaxation of gastroesophageal sphincter o Decreased intestinal motility o Stasis of contents of gallbladder o Increase in biliary cholesterol content
NO: nitric oxide

Ans: (c) ALP

Ref: *DC Dutta Obstetrics, 9th edition, Page 51*

5. False statement regarding chorionic villous sampling:

(a) Chorionic villous sampling done at 16-21 weeks

(b) Done for chromosomal abnormality

(c) Increased nuchal Translucency indication for chorionic villous sampling

(d) Trophoblastic cells are tested

Explanation:

Chorionic Villous Sampling (CVS)

- Is done for prenatal diagnosis of genetic disorders
- It is carried out between **10-13 weeks transcervically** and **transabdominally** from **10 weeks to term.**
- It is done under USG guidance with the help of the long polyethylene catheter with a metal obturator
- 15-25 mg of villi is aspirated.
- Transabdominally spinal needle of 18-20 gauge is used.
- Karyotype result comes in 24 hours in direct preparation and tissue culture takes 10-14 days
- **Complications** include:
  - **Fetal loss (1-2%)**
  - Oromandibular deformity
  - Limb deformity

- Chromosomal anomalies like Down's syndrome, Turner's syndrome and single gene disorders like cystic fibrosis, taysachs disease ca be diagnosed using CVS.

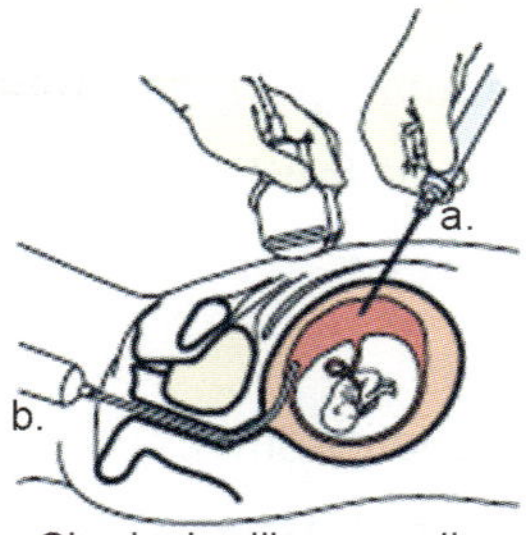

Chorionic villus sampling
a. Transabdominal b. Transvaginal

Prenatal invasive diagnostic procedures			
	Chorionic villus sampling	**Amniocentesis**	**Fetal blood sampling**
Gestational age	First trimester (after 10 weeks)	After 15 weeks	After 18 weeks
Route	Transabdominal/transcervical	Transabdominal	Transabodominal
Site of sampling	Thickest part of placenta	Most accessible pocket of fluid	Umbilical cord/ intrahepatic portal vein/ fetal heart
Tissue obtained	Placental villi	Amniotic fluid (amniocytes)	Fetal blood (RBCs, serum)
Time taken to obtain karyotyping	• Metaphase culture: 1-3 weeks • Fish: 48-72 hours	• Metaphase culture: 1-3 weeks • Fish: 48-72 hours	48-72 hours
Risk of pregnancy loss	0.5-1%	0.5-1%	<2%
FISH: Fluorescence in situ hybridization; *RBCs:* Red Blood Cells.			

Ans: (a) Chorionic villous sampling done at 16-21 weeks

Ref: *DC Dutta, Obstetrics, 9th edition, Page 105*

6. Uteroplacental blood flow per minute:

(a) 200 ml / minute
(b) 500 ml / minute
(c) 300 ml / minute
(d) 600-700 ml / minute

Explanation:

- Volume of blood in mature placenta – **500 ml**
- Volume of blood in intervillous space – **150 ml**
- Blood flow in the intervillous space – **600-700 ml/min**
- Fetal blood flow through the placenta – **400 ml/min**

Ans: (d) 600-700 ml/min

Ref: *DC Dutta, Obstetrics, 9th edition, Page 28*

7. Regarding Listeriosis in pregnancy, which of the following is false?

(a) Cause 2nd trimester loss
(b) Infection on drinking raw milk
(c) Symptoms occur after 3 days of exposure
(d) Leads to granulomatosis infantiseptica

Explanation:

Listeriosis

- Listeria monocytogenes is an **intra-cellular gram positive bacillus.**
- Infection is caused by consuming **infected food** or contact with **infected products of animals (milk)**.
- Incubation period is on an **average 30 days.**
- **Symptoms –** Flu like or food poisoning.
- **Investigations –** Blood culture during septicaemia.
- **Complications – Late miscarriage (2nd trimester), preterm labour, still birth, meningitis, encephalitis, pneumonia, gastroenteritis and neonatal death.**
- **Treatment –** Ampicillin, amoxycillin, gentamycin, cotrimoxazole.
- Prevention – Avoiding drinking unpasteurized milk, soft cheese, refrigerated smoked sea food.
- Surviving neonates of fetomaternal listeriosis may suffer **granulomatosis infantiseptica** — pyogenic granulomas distributed over the whole body.

Ans: (c) Symptoms occur after 3 days of exposure

Ref: *DC Dutta, Obstetrics, 9th edition, Page 278*

8. Fetal blood flow through placenta:

(a) 200 ml/min (b) 400 ml/min
(c) 900 ml/min (d) 100 ml/min

Explanation:

- Fetal blood flow through placenta **400 ml/min**
- Blood flow through intervillous space **600-700 ml/min**
- Pressure in the intervillous space during contraction (30-40 mm Hg) and during relaxation (10-15 mm Hg)
- Pressure in the uterine artery **70-80 mm Hg**
- Pressure in the uterine vein **8 mm Hg**
- Pressure in the umbilical artery **60 mm Hg**
- Pressure in the umbilical vein **10 mm Hg**
- Fetal capillary pressure in villi **20-40 mm Hg**

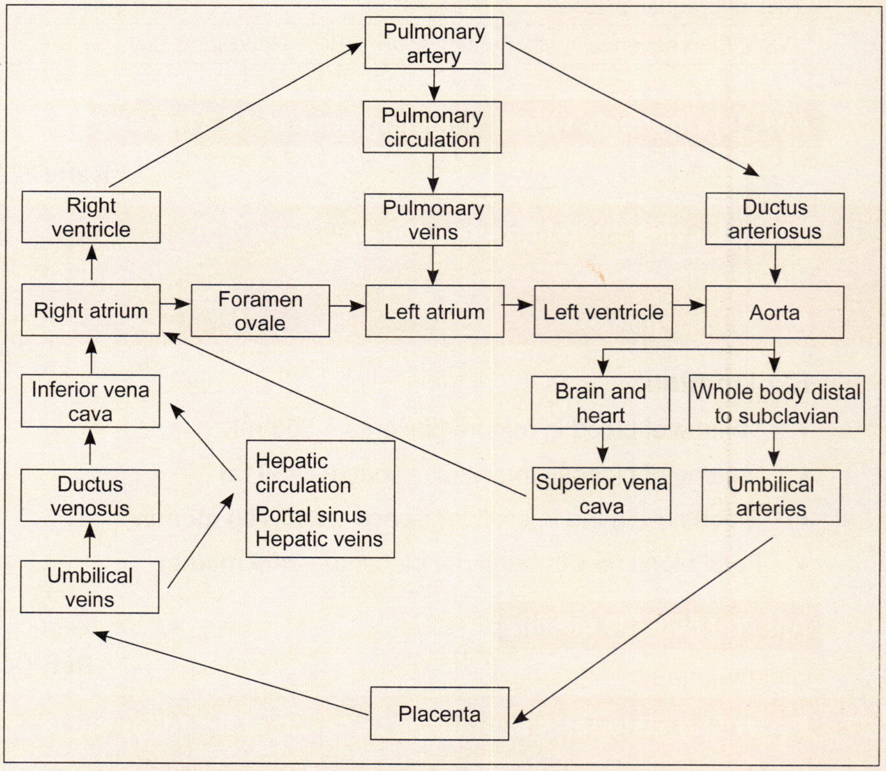

Figure: The fetal circulation, a schematic representation

Ans: (b) 400 ml/min

Ref: *DC Dutta, Obstetrics, 9th edition, Page 28*

9. A 19 years pregnant woman with mitral valve area 1.4 sq cm is admitted at 6 weeks. She is on antiarrhythmic drugs. Presently she is in NYHA2. She was diagnosed with RHD with MS at 16 years age. What is the risk of maternal mortality?

(a) <1% (b) 50%

(c) 15% (d) 5%

Explanation:

Risk categorization of cardiac disease in pregnancy	
Risk category	**Cardiac disease**
Low risk (maternal mortality <1%)	• Septal defects • Mitral stenosis, NYHA class I and class II • Patent ductus arteriosus • Pulmonary/tricuspid lesions
Moderate risk (maternal mortality 5%-15%)	• Mitral stenosis, NYHA class III and class IV • Marfan syndrome with normal aorta • Uncomplicated coarctation of aorta • Uncorrected TOF • Prosthetic valves
High risk (maternal mortality 25%-50%)	• Eisenmenger syndrome • Pulmonary hypertension • Marfan syndrome with abnormal aorta • Dilated cardiomyopathy

NYHA: New York Heart Association; TOF: Tetralogy of Fallot

Factors increasing risk of pulmonary edema

- Normal pregnancy
  - Pregnancy at 28-30 weeks when blood volume peaks
  - Labor
    - Due to pumping of blood from uterus
  - Immediate postpartum
    - Due to shunting of blood from placental bed
  - Puerperium
    - Due to mobilization of extravascular fluid
- Intercurrent events
  - Hypertension
  - Anemia
  - Multifetal pregnancy
  - Thyrotoxicosis
  - Acute febrile illness
  - Atrial fibrillation

Ans: (a) < 1%

Ref: *DC Dutta, Obstetrics, 9th edition, Page 258*

10. Which trophoblast takes part in invasion of arteriole?

(a) Tertiary (b) Interstitial

(c) Endovascular (d) Extravillous

Explanation:

- The **cytotrophoblast** that lines the **villous stems** are called **villous cytotrophoblast***.
- The cytotrophoblast which **invades the decidua** are known as **interstitial extravillous cytotrophoblast***.
- The cytotrophoblast that invades the **spiral arteries** are known as **intravascular/endovascular extravillous cytotrophoblast***.

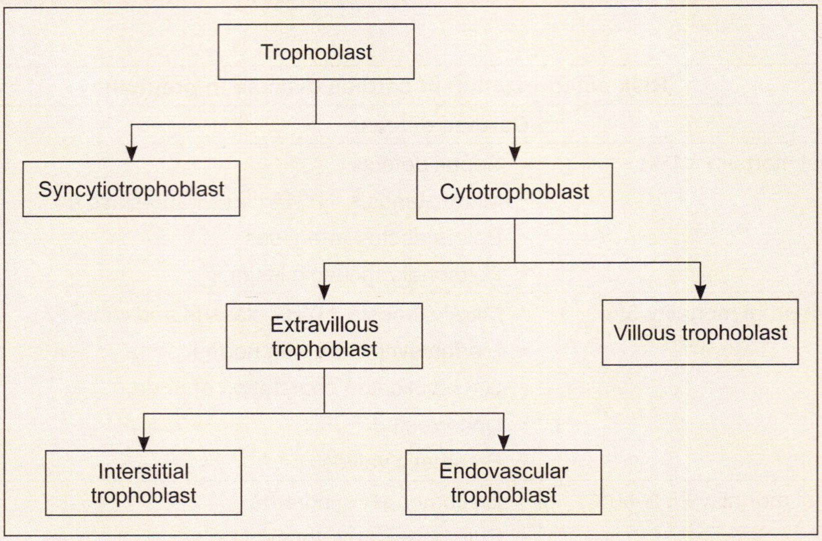

Figure: Differentiation of trophoblast

Extravillous trophoblastic invasion
• Interstitial trophoblast ○ Invades decidua basalis and myometrium ○ Forms placental bed giant cells • Endovascular trophoblast ○ Invades spiral arteries – First phase (by 12 weeks): Invades arteries in decidua – Second phase (by 16 weeks): Invades arteries in myometrium

Functions of the trophoblasts
• Syncytiotrophoblast ○ Transports nutrients and gases ○ Secretes peptide and steroid hormones • Villous trophoblast ○ Formation of villi ○ Transports of nutrients and gases • Interstitial trophoblast ○ Interacts with cells of maternal immune system • Endovascular trophoblast ○ Facilitates placental blood flow

Ans: (c) Endovascular

Ref: *DC Dutta, Obstetrics, 9th edition, Page 21*

11. Drugs that have been under "FDA-X" category in pregnancy/which of the following is a category X drug?

(a) Itraconazole
(b) Isotretinoin
(c) Misoprostol
(d) Cyclophosphamide

Explanation:

- **Category X** drugs are **contraindicated** in pregnancy
- Proven fetal risk clearly outway any possible benefit
- **Drugs in this group are:**
  - Alcohol

- ACE inhibitors
- Lithium
- Methotrexate
- Valproic acid
- Mifepristone
- Danazol
- Isotretinoin
- Radioactive iodine

Critical periods (weeks of gestation) of susceptibility for different fetal organs
• Heart: 3-4 • Limbs: 4.5-7.5 • Eyes: 4.5-8.5 • Ears: 4.5-9.5 • External genitalia: 8-9 • Brain and skeletal system: Beginning of week 3 to end of pregnancy

Safety rating system for drugs
Category A: Safety established • Controlled studies in women show no risk to fetus in first trimester • No evidence of risk in later trimesters • Possibility of fetal harm appears remote *Category B: Safety likely* • Animal studies show to fetal risk but no controlled studies in pregnant women *or* • Animal studies have shown adverse effect but not confirmed in women in first or later trimesters *Category C: Teratogenicity possible* • Studies in animals have revealed adverse effects on the fetus (teratogenic, embryoidal, or other) but no controlled studies in women *or* • Studies in women and animals not available • These drugs should be given only if the potential benefit justifies the potential risk to the fetus *Category D: Teratogenicity probable* • Positive evidence of human fetal risk, but the benefits from use in pregnant women may be acceptable despite the risk, if the drug is needed in: ○ A life-threatening situation *or* ○ A serious disease for which safter drugs cannot be used or are ineffective *Category X: Teratogenicity likely* • Studies in animals and humans have demonstrated fetal abnormalities and/or • There is evidence of fetal risk based on human experience *and* • The risk of the use of the drug in pregnant women clearty outweighs any possible benefit • Contraindicated in women who are or may become pregnant

Some teratogenic prescription drugs (Category X)
• Androgens and testosterone derivatives (e.g., danazol) • Angiotensin-converting enzyme (ACE) inhibitors (e.g., enalapril, captopril) and angiotensin II receptor blockers • Coumadin derivatives (e.g., warfarin) • Carbamazepine

Contd.

Contd.

- Diethylstilbestrol
- Folic acid antagonists (methotrexate and aminopterin)
- Lithium
- Phenytoin
- Primidone
- Statins
- Streptomycin and kanamycin
- Tetracycline
- Thalidomide and leflunomide
- Trimethadione and paramethadione
- Valproic acid
- Vitamin A above recommended daily allowance (RDA), and its derivatives (e.g., isotretinoin, etretinate, and retinoids)

Ans: (b) Isotretinoin

Ref: *DC Dutta Obstetrics, 9th edition, Page 475*

12. Most common site for fibroids in uterus is:

(a) Subserous (b) Intramural

(c) Subserous (d) Cervical

Explanation:

Uterine Fibroids

- Fibroids are the **most common** benign solid tumours in **females.**
- Most common tumour of uterus.
- Fibroids are **estrogen dependent** for growth.
- **Progesterone inhibits** their **growth.**
- **GnRH shrinks size** of **fibroid.**
- **Increases in size** during **pregnancy** and **OCP intake.**
- **Decreases** in size after **menopause.**
- The presence of **myoma** causes **hyperplasia** of the **myometrial wall.**
- The cavity of the uterus is often distorted and enlarged.
- The **endometrium** tends to be **thicker** due to **endometrial hyperplasia.**
- The ovaries at times are **enlarged,** cystic and hyperaemic with evidence of **salpingo-oophoritis** in about **15%** cases.
- Distribution of fibroid in the body of uterus:
  - **Intramural – 75% (Most common)**
  - **Submucus – 15%**
  - **Subserous – 10%**
- Most **common site** is **body of uterus*.**
- A typical myoma is a well-circumscribed tumour with a **pseudocapsule.**
- The vessels which supply blood to the tumour lie in the capsule and send radial branches into the tumour.

Because of this arrangement of blood supply, the **central portion of the tumour** receives the **least blood supply,** and **degeneration** is noticeable early and most often in this part of the tumour. On the other hand, **calcification begins at the periphery** and spreads inwards along the vessels.

- Microscopically, the tumour consists of **bundles of plain muscle cells,** separated by varying amount of fibrous strands. Areas of embryonic muscle tissue may be present in a myoma.
- The endometrium tends to be thicker due to **endometrial hyperplasia.** The ovaries at times are enlarged, cystic and hyperaemic with evidence of **salpingo-oophoritis in about 15%** cases.

ALSO NOTE:

- Most common complication of fibroid during **pregnancy – Red degeneration.**
- Incidence of **sarcomatous** change in fibroid – **0.5%.**
- Most common presenting symptom is menorrhagia.
- **Metrorrhagia** is caused by **– submucus fibroid.**
- Most common **degeneration – Hyaline** degeneration.
- Recurrent pregnancy loss is associated with **submucous fibroid**.
- **Polycythemia** in **myoma** is due to **extramedullary erythropoisis** within the substance of **myoma.**
- **Danazole, GnRH** and **RU 486 reduces** the **size of fibroids.**

Ans: (b) Intramural

Ref: *Shaw's Textbook of Gynaecology, 15th edition, Page 352*

13. Schiller duval bodies are seen in:

(a) Endodermal sinus tumour
(b) Embryonal carcinoma
(c) Dermoid cyst
(d) Brenner tumour

Explanation:

- **Schiller duval bodies** are characteristic histological feature of **endodermal sinus tumour.**
- They are tuft of vascular tissue inside cystic spaces lined by flattened epithelium.

Endodermal Sinus Tumour

- Originate from **multipotential embryonal tissue** as a result of selective differentiation of yolk sac structures
- Peak - 15 to 20 years of age
- Second most common malignant germ cell tumour of ovary
- Unilateral, solid, >10 cms diameter
- **Micro-schiller duval bodies,** eosinophilic hyaline bodies containing alpha protein
- Associated with **dysgerminoma**
- Treatment–Surgical staging and unilateral salpingo-oopherectomy
- **Combination chemotherapy–POMB-ACE regimen** (cyclophosphamide, vincristine, methotrexate, bleomycin, actinomycin D, cisplatin, etoposide) **VAC regimen, VBP regimen.**
- Tumor marker–**alpha fetoprotein >20 microgm/ml,** Elevated **alpha 1 antitrypsin.**
- Respond well to chemotherapy and good survival rate.

Ans: (a) Endodermal sinus tumour

Ref: *Dutta, Textbook of Gynecology, 5th edition, Page 368*

ORTHOPEDICS

1. Kohler's disease affects:

(a) Calcaneum
(b) Tarsal bone
(c) Talus
(d) Humerus-Capitulum

Explanation:

- **Kohler's disease** is osteochondritis of **navicular*** (**tarsal bone).**

Some Other Important Osteochondritis Names to Remember:

- **Keinbock's disease**–Lunate
- **Freiberg's disease**–Metatarsal heads
- **Panner's disease**–Capitullum
- **Scheurman's disease**–Ring epiphysis of vertebrae
- **Calve's disease**–Central bony nucleus of vertebrae
- **Tibial tuberosity**–Osgood-Schlatter
- **Calcaneal epiphysis**–Severe's disease
- **Lower pole of patella**–Johanssen-Larsen syndrome

Ans: (b) Tarsal bone

Ref: *Fundamentals of Orthopedics by Mohindra and Jain, 2nd edition, Jaypee Publishers, Page 443*

2. Lisfranc fracture dislocation involves:

(a) Lunate
(b) Scaphoid
(c) Trans-metatarsal
(d) Capitate

Explanation:

- **The Lisfranc joint** consists of the **tarsometatarsal joint complex**, which includes the **three cuneiforms**, **cuboid** and their articulations with the **five metatarsal bones.**
- Dislocations of the **Lisfranc joint** are the **most common dislocations of the foot**.

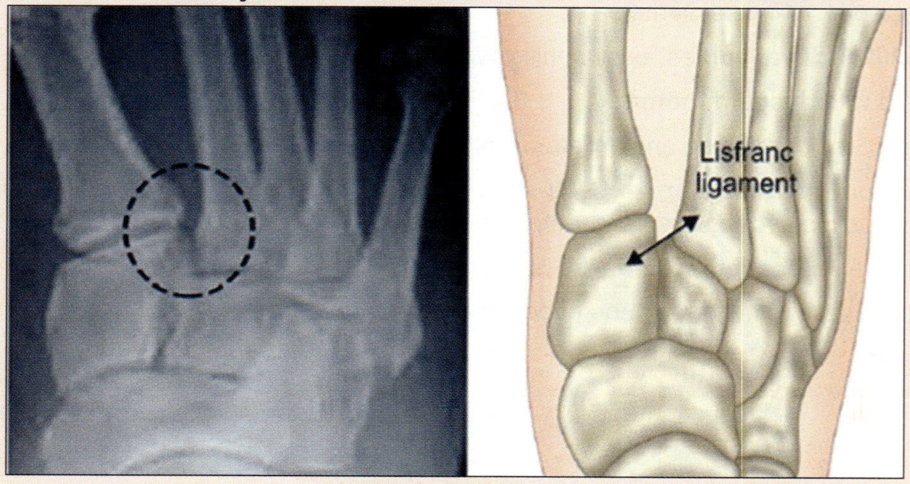

Figure: Lisfranc dislocation

- These injuries usually result from high-energy injuries like forced hyperflexion in road traffic accidents and fall from height.

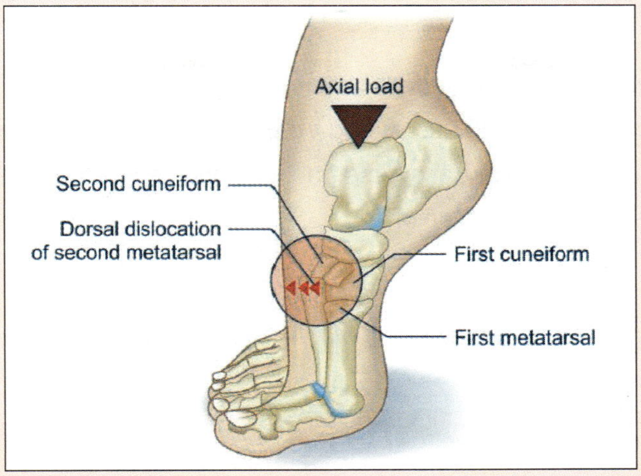

Figure: Mechanism of Lisfranc fracture dislocation (taken from Fundamentals of Orthopedics)

Ans: (c) Trans-metatarsal

Ref: *Fundamentals of Orthopedics by Mohindra and Jain, 2nd edition, Jaypee Publishers, Page 160*

3. Examine the given X-ray picture. What is the diagnosis?

(a) Bucket handle fracture (b) Malgaigne fracture
(c) Straddle fracture (d) Sacro iliac joint dislocation

Explanation:

- Image shows fracture of **ipsilateral pubic rami** and **ilium** (near the SI joint) which is characteristic of **Malgaigne's fracture**.

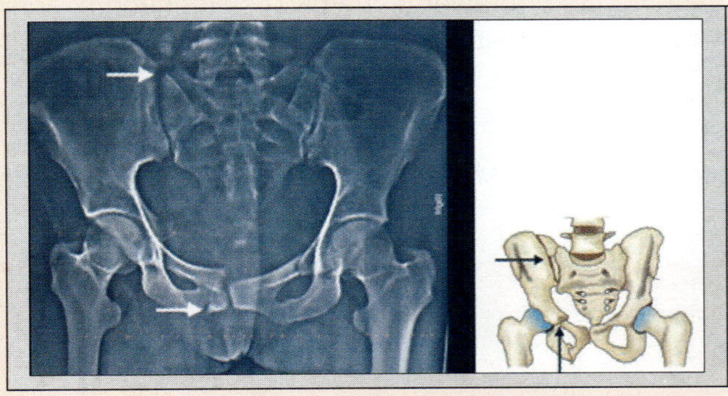

Figure: Malgaigne's fracture

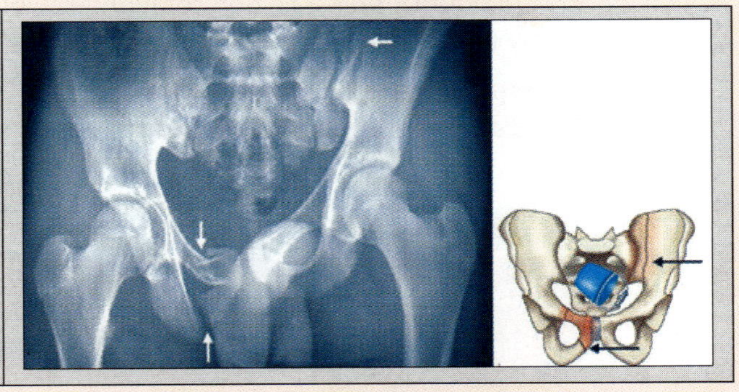

Figure: Bucket handle fracture

Ans: (b) Malgaigne fracture

Ref: *Fundamentals of Orthopedics by Mohindra and Jain, 2nd edition, Jaypee Publishers, Page 115*

4. Which fracture is caused by fall on ground with flexed wrist?

(a) Colles # (b) Chauffeur fracture
(c) Barton # (d) Smith #

Explanation:

- **Smith's fracture** is **reverse Colles fracture** and is caused by a fall on the **dorsal aspect of the hand (flexed hand)**.

Smith Fractures (also known as **Goyrand fractures)**

- Fractures of the **distal radius** with associated **volar angulation** of the **distal fracture fragment(s)**.
- These fractures are extra-articular transverse fractures and can be thought of as a reverse Colles fracture.
- Garden spade deformity due to malunion.

Ans: (d) Smith #

Ref: *Fundamentals of Orthopedics by Mohindra and Jain, 2nd edition, Jaypee Publishers, Page 94*

5. All are seen in anterior cruciate ligament (ACL) tear except:

(a) Anterior dislocation of tibia
(b) Segond fracture
(c) Deep intercondylar fossa
(d) High tibial slope

Explanation:

- **Narrow (not wide/deep) intercondylar notch*** may predispose to ACL injury by causing impingement.
- **Segond fracture*** is an avulsion fracture of the knee that involves the lateral aspect of the tibial plateau and is very frequently (~75% of cases) associated with disruption of the anterior cruciate ligament (ACL).

Anterior Cruciate Ligament

- **Lachman's test** (most sensitive done at 20° knee flexion).
- **Anterior drawer** test (done at 90° of knee flexion).
- **Pivot shift test**/flexion rotation drawer test (2nd best).
- Test for ACL in decreasing order of sensitivity and specificity:
  - Lachman's test > flexion rotation drawer test > anterior drawer test > pivot shift phenomenon tested by lateral pivot shift test of macintosh or jerk test of Hughston and loose.

Ans: (c) Deep intercondylar fossa

Ref: *Geng B et al. Chin Med J (Engl.) 2016 Nov 5;129(21):2540-45*

6. Incorrect statement regarding Jefferson fracture:

(a) Fracture of C1 vertebra
(b) Caused by fall of heavy weight on head
(c) Is associated with high mortality
(d) Involves both anterior and posterior ring of atlas

Explanation:

- At **C1** level only **35%** of the canal is occupied by the cord with plenty of space as opposed to 50% occupancy in the lower spine, hence, neurologic injury is uncommon.

Jefferson's Fracture

- Jefferson fracture is burst fracture of **ring of atlas (CI) vertebrae.**
- Burst fracture is a **vertical compression** fracture.
- Mechanism: Axial blow to head.

- Involves both anterior and posterior ring of atlas.
- Though a serious injury, the long-term consequences of a Jefferson's fracture are uncertain and may not impact longevity or abilities, even if untreated.

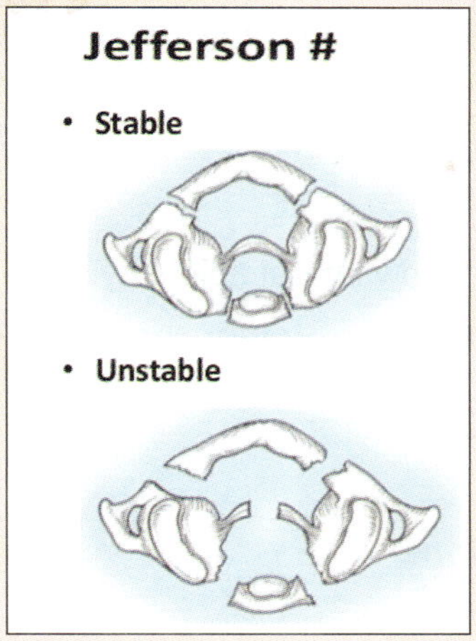

Ans: (c) Is associated with high mortality

Ref: *Fundamentals of Orthopedics by Mohindra and Jain, 2nd edition, Jaypee Publishers, Page 221*

7. Middle finger extension test (Maudsley test) is done for:

(a) Medial epicondylitis
(b) Carpal tunnel syndrome
(c) Lateral epicondylitis
(d) Dequervain's disease

Explanation:

- **Maudsley's test:** Pain in the region of the lateral epicondyle during resisted extension of the middle finger.

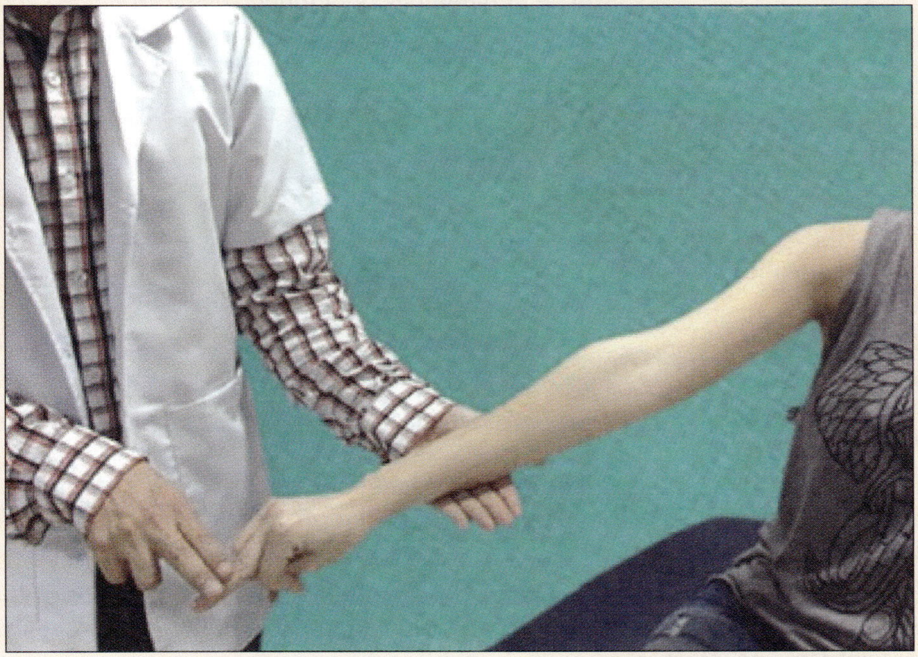

Figure: Maudsley's test for Tennis elbow/Lateral epicondylitis (taken from Fundamentals of Orthopedics)

TENNIS ELBOW/LATERAL EPICONDYLITIS

- It is chronic tendonitis of **common extensor origin** (especially **extensor carpi radialis brevis**) on **lateral epicondyle**.
- It may result in **small tears**, **fibrocartilaginous metaplasia**, **microscopic calcification** and **painful vascular reaction** in tendon fibers close to lateral epicondyle (degenerative changes with **angiofibroblastic proliferation).**

Clinical Features

- **Localized tenderness** at or just below lateral epicondyle.
- Pain can be demonstrated by passively **stretching** the **extensor radialis brevis**; this is done by extending the elbow, pronating the forearm and then passively flexing the wrist or active extension of wrist against resistance can produce pain (**Cozen's test***).
- **Treatment** includes:
  - **Anti-inflammatory medications.**
  - **Steroid injection.**
  - Detachment of common extensor origin, orbicular ligament and synovial fringe.

Also Note:

- **Golfer's Elbow Medial epicondylitis** involving common **flexor pronator origin.**
- **Baseball Pitcher's Elbow**, repetitive, vigorous throwing activities can cause damage to the bones or soft tissue attachment around elbow. Hypertrophy of lower humerus and incongruity of the joint, or loose body formation and osteoarthritis.
- The junior equivalent (**Little leaguer's elbow**) is a partial avulsion of **medial epicondyle**.
- **Javelin Thrower's Elbow:** It is avulsion of **tip of Olecranon** due to over arm action.

Ans: (c) Lateral epicondylitis

Ref: *Fundamentals of Orthopedics by Mohindra and Jain, 2nd edition, Jaypee Publishers, Page 175*

8. Monteggia fracture is due to:

(a) Proximal third of ulna fracture and radial head dislocation
(b) Distal third of radius fracture and ulnar head dislocation
(c) Proximal radial fracture and ulnar head dislocation
(d) Distal ulnar fracture and radial head dislocation

Explanation:

Monteggia Fracture

- The injury described by Monteggia in the early nineteenth century was a **fracture** of the shaft of the **proximal third of ulna** associated with **dislocation of the proximal radioulnar joint**. The radiocapitellar joint is dislocated as well.
- More recently, the definition has been extended to embrace almost **any fracture of the ulna** associated with **dislocation of the radio-capitellar joint**, including transolecranon fractures in which the proximal radioulnar joint remains intact.
- If the ulnar shaft fracture is angulated with the apex anterior (**the most common type**) then the radial head is displaced anteriorly, if the fracture apex is posterior, the radial dislocation is **posterior**, and if the fracture apex is **lateral** then the radial head will be **laterally** displaced.

- In **children**, the ulnar injury may be an **incomplete fracture** (**greenstick or plastic deformation of the shaft**).
- Fractures of the **distal third of radius** with **dislocation of the ulnar head from the distal radioulnar joint** was described by **Galeazzi** in 1934 and named after him. It is commoner than Monteggia fracture dislocation.

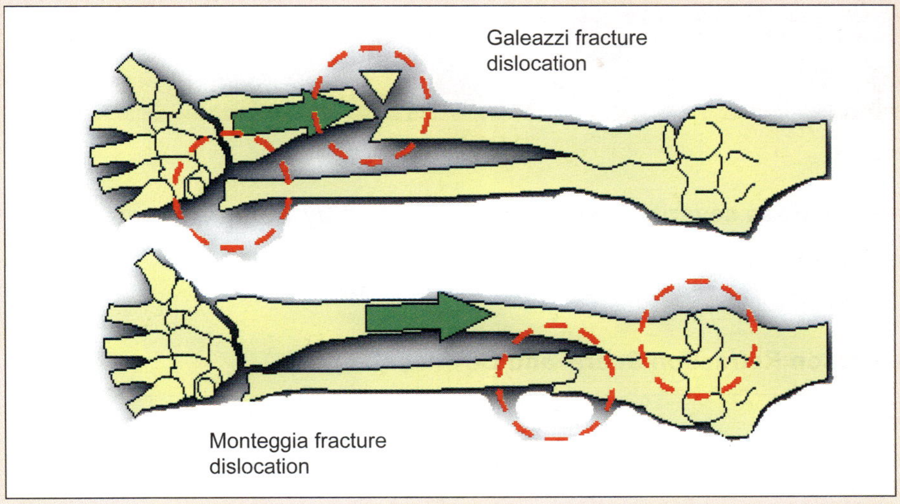

Ans: (a) Proximal third of ulna fracture and radial head dislocation

Ref: *Apley's System of Orthopaedics and Fractures, 9th edition, Page 770 & 773*

PEDIATRICS

1. Which of the following scoring is done to assess respiratory distress in Neonates?

(a) CRIB score
(b) APGAR score
(c) Silverman-Anderson score
(d) SNAP score

Explanation:

The respiratory distress severity in neonate is assessed by 2 scoring systems:

- Silverman-Anderson Retraction Score and
- Downes Score

Silverman-Anderson Retraction Score and Downes Score:

Score	0	1	2
Silverman-Anderson Retraction Score			
Upper chest retraction	Synchronised	Lag on inspiration	See-Saw breathing
Lower chest retraction	None	Just visible	Marked
Xiphoid retraction	None	Just visible	Marked
Nasal dilatation	None	Minimal	Marked
Grunt	None	Heard with stethoscope	Heard without stethoscope
Downes Score			
Respiratory rate	<60 per minute	60 – 80 per minute	> 80 per minute
Cyanosis	Absent in room air	In room air	In FiO_2 > 40%
Air entry	Normal	Mild decrease	Barely auduible
Grunt	None	Heard with stethoscope	Heard without stethoscope
Retraction	Nil	Mild	Moderate to severe

- Score should be monitored every 30 minutes to 1 hour to monitor for progression of respiratory distress.
- Progressive FiO_2 requirement to maintain SpO_2 (90 – 92%) in preterm and (94 – 96%) in term neonate is a sensitive indicator of severe distress.
- Indications for starting **CPAP*** are a Downes or Silverman score of **>6 at birth** or a FiO_2 requirement of **>0.4** to maintain an acceptable saturation on pulse oximeter.

Option A – CRIB (Clinical Risk Index for Babies) Scoring System

1. Predicts initial risk of mortality amongst the low birth weight babies.
2. **Factors** – Birth weight, Gestational age, Congenital malformations, Maximum base escess in first 12 hours, Minimum appropriate FiO_2 in first 12 hours, Maximum appropriate FiO_2 in first 12 hours.
3. **CRIB II** – Factors – gender, gestational age, birth weight, admission temperature and base excess.
4. **Other scoring systems**: Berlin score, National Therapeutic Intervention Scoring System (NTISS), National Institute of Child Health and Human Development (NICHHD).

Option B – APGAR Score

Apgar score at birth and 1 min after birth was initially developed to assess:

- Immediate condition of the newborn and
- Potential need for resuscitation.

Apgar Scoring System			
Sign	**0**	**1**	**2**
A ppearance (color)	Blue / Pale	Pink body, Blue extremities	All pink
P ulse (heart) rate	Absent	<100 per minute	>100 per minute
G rimace (Reflex irritability)	No response	Grimace	Cough / sneeze
A ttitude (tone)	Limp	Some flexion of extremities	Active motion
R espiratory effort	Absent	Slow (irregular)	Good crying

Option D: SNAP Score (Score for Neonatal Acute Physiology) Score.

1. A physiology based illness severity score based on measurements of 28 items collected over the first 24 hours of life.
2. **SNAP – PE** (Score for Neonatal Acute Physiology – **Perinatal Extension**) – Contains the 28 SNAP parameters along with 3 factors (birth weight, APGAR < 7 at 5 minutes and small for gestation age).
3. **SNAP – II:** A six item score based on variables collected during the first 12 hours after admission.
4. **SNAP– PE – II:** SNAP II + (birth weight < 749 gm, APGAR < 7 at 5 minutes and small for gestation age).

EXTRA EDGE:

- **Silverman-Anderson Retraction Score** – More suited for **preterm** with **Hyaline Membrane Disease** while.
- **Downes Score** – Can be applied to any gestational age and respiratory condition.

Ans: (c) Silverman-Anderson score

Ref: *Dorling JS, Field DJ, Manktelow B, Neonatal Disease Severity Scoring Systems Archives of Disease in Childhood – Fetal and Neonatal, edition 2005;90:F11-F16*

2. A neonate's blood culture grows extended spectrum beta-lactamase (ESBL) organism. All will be the correct empirical therapy in this situation except:

(a) Piperacillin tazobactum
(b) Meropenam
(c) Astreonam
(d) Cefotetan

Explanation:

- Extended spectrum beta-lactamases (ESBLs) – by definition are resistant to **betalactum antibiotics** like **monobactams (Astreonam, Tigemonam, Carumona and Nocardicin A).**

Extended Spectrum Beta-Lactamases (ESBLs)

- ESBLs are defined as enzymes produced by certain bacteria that are able to hydrolyze ***extended spectrum cephalosporin (ceftazidime, ceftriaxone, cefotaxime and monobactam).***
- **Klebsiella pneumoniae** and **E. coli** are most frequently associated with ESBL production.
- All clinically significant isolates of E. coli or K. pneumoniae should be tested against betalactam drugs either using a disc diffusion method or the minimum inhibition concentration (MIC) method.
- Any decrease in the zone sizes or MIC **less than 2 mg/L for the 3rd generation cephalosporins** should be used as a criterion to test for ESBLs.

- ***Carbapenems*** (Imipenem, Meropenem, Etrapenem and Doripenam), ***cephamycine*** (Cefoxitin, Cefotetan, Cefmetazole) and ***piperacillin/tazobactam*** are currently most effective against ESBL producer strains.

Carbapenem Resistance:

- Carbapenem resistance occur in **gram-negative** organisms by either:
  - The acquisition of **specific enzymes** such as the **transposon-mediated Klebsiella pneumoniae carbapenemase (KPC**), OR
  - By **reduced carbapenem influx** caused by the loss of outer membrane protein porin in ESBL organisms.
- The modified Hodge test is recommended for carbapenemase surveillance.
  - Current treatment (with most carbapenemase-producing organisms).
  - Requires the use of the ***polymyxin B***, an antibiotic with significantly toxicity.

EXTRA EDGE:

- The most important beta-lactamase that is prevalent is **TEM-1.**
- Another prevalent type of beta-lactamases is **SHV-1** (responsible for plasmid mediated ampicillin resistance in bacteria which harbors it).

Ans: (c) Astreonam

Ref: *Manual of Neonatal Care (John P. Cloherty), 7th edition, Page 641*

3. All the following are causes of hypotonia in a 2-year-old child except:

(a) Trisomy 21
(b) Spinal muscular atrophy
(c) Congenital muscular dystrophy
(d) Cerebral palsy

Explanation:

- All the above causes presents exclusively with **hypotonia** (either central or peripheral), except for **cerebral palsy (CP).**
- Cerebral palsy commonly presents with **hypertonia**, though **hypotonic CP** is a known entity; its occurrence is uncommon than hypertonic CP.

Difference between central and peripheral hypotonia:

Factors	Central Hypotonia	Peripheral Hypotonia
Reflex	• Increased	• Hypo / Areflexia
Plantar Response	• Extensor	• No Response
Clonus	• Present	• Absent
Developmental Delay	• Global	• Selective with Preserved Social Interaction
Head Circumference	• Microcephaly	• Normal For Age
Weakness	• Axial Muscles	• Anti-Gravitational Limb Muscles
Convulsions	• Present	• Absent
Fasciculations/atrophy	• Absent	• Present
Causes	• Trisomy 21 • Prader Willi Syndrome • Zellweger Syndrome • Cerebral malformations • Hypoxic Ischaemic Encephalopathy	• Poliomyelitis • Guillain-Barré syndrome • Myasthenia Gravis • Botulism • Spinal Muscular Atrophy • Congenital Myotonic Dystrophy • Congenital Structural Myopathies

Contd.

Contd.

Investigations	• Karyotyping • Very long chain fatty acid assay • Neuroimaging – CT / MRI	• Mutation analysis • Muscle or Nerve Biopsy • Nerve Conduction studies • Electro Myogram • Creatinine Kinase levels

EXTRA EDGE:

- Hypotonia with profound **weakness** sugests **LMN lesion.**
- Hypotonia with **preserved power** (except in acute stage) suggests **UMN lesion**.
- **Hypotonic Cerebral palsy** – Rare subtype of CP which presents with **hyotonia***.

Ans: (d) Cerebral palsy

Ref: *Van Toorn R. Clinical Approach to the Floppy Child, CME, 2004;22:449–55*

4. Which of the following malignancy is seen in male child with short stature, low IQ, murmur in pulmonary area and lymphedema?

(a) Retinoblastoma (b) Hepatocellular carcinoma

(c) Juvenile myelomonocytic leukemia (d) Germ cell tumour

Explanation:

- ***Male child with short stature***, low IQ, ***murmur in pulmonary area*** and ***lymphedema*** suggests Noonan syndrome with pulmonary valve stenosis.
- **Hematological abnormality seen in** Noonan syndrome **is Juvenile Myelomonocytic Leukemia.**

Noonan Syndrome:

- Autosomal dominant disorder resulting from mutations [RAS-MAPK (mitogen-activated protein kinase) pathway.
- The most common of these is *PTPN11* (encodes a protein-tyrosine phosphatase (SHP-2) on chromosome 12q24.1).

Features of Noonan Syndrome:

- **Short stature**
- Failure to thrive (use Noonan growth curve)
- Tall forehead with epicanthal folds/Ptosis/Blue-green irises/Hypertelorism
- Low nasal bridge, upturned nose
- Downward-slanting palpebral fissures/Myopia/Nystagmus
- Low-set auricles
- Low posterior hairline
- **Short webbed neck** (excessive nuchal skin), **cystic hygroma**
- **Shield chest**/Pectus carinatum superiorly
- Pigmented villonodular synovitis (polyarticular)/Cubitus valgus
- **Pulmonary valve stenosis** (dysplastic valve)
- **Hypertrophic cardiomyopathy / Atrial Septal Defect**
- Lymphedema / Nevi, lentigines, café-au-lait spots
- **Cryptorchidism / Small penis / Delayed puberty**

- **Amegakaryocytic thrombocytopenia** as well as pancytopenia with a hypocellular marrow.
- Leukemia, myeloproliferative disorder.

They share many clinical features with Turner syndrome (old name was **pseudo-Turner syndrome)**

In contrast to Turner syndrome:

Noonan syndrome
- Affects both sexes; and
- Different pattern of congenital heart disease, typically involving right-sided lesions (pulmonary valve).

Conditions having familial susceptibility for malignancy:

Disorder	Malignancy
• **Chromosome 11p deletion syndrome**	• Wilms tumor
• **Chromosome 13q deletion syndrome**	• Retinoblastoma • Sarcoma
• **Trisomy 21**	• Megakaryocytic leukemia • Transient leukemoid reaction
• **Klinefelter syndrome (47,XXY)**	• Breast cancer • Extragonadal germ cell tumors
• **Trisomy 8**	• Preleukemia
• ***Noonan syndrome***	• ***Juvenile myelomonocytic leukemia***
• **Shwachman-Diamond syndrome**	• Acute Myeloid Leukemia
• **Diamond-Blackfan anemia**	• Acute Myeloid Leukemia • Myelodysplastic syndrome • Osteogenic sarcoma
• **Hemochromatosis** • **Glycogen storage disease 1 (von Gierke disease)** • **Tyrosinemia** • **Galactosemia**	• Hepatocellular carcinoma
• **Turcot syndrome**	• Pediatric brain tumors
• **Familial adenomatous polyposis**	• Colorectal carcinoma • Thyroid carcinoma, • Duodenal carcinoma • Periampullar carcinomas
• **von Hippel-Lindau disease**	• Hemangioblastoma of the cerebellum and retina • Pheochromocytoma
• **Gorlin-Goltz syndrome (nevus basal cell carcinoma syndrome)**	• Multiple basal cell carcinomas • Medulloblastoma
• **X-linked immunodeficiency (Duncan syndrome)** • **Wiskott-Aldrich syndrome** • **X-linked agammaglobulinemia (Bruton disease)** • **Severe combined immunodeficiency** • **Ataxia-telangiectasia** • **Bloom syndrome** • **Fanconi anemia**	• Lymphoma • Leukemia
• **Xeroderma pigmentosum**	• Basal cell and squamous cell carcinomas • Melanoma

Ans: (c) Juvenile mono-myelocytic leukemia

Ref: *Nelson Textbook of Pediatrics, 20th edition, Page 2420*

5. Which epileptic syndrome is associated with left hemispheric atrophy in child?

(a) Dravet Syndrome
(b) Dyke Davidson Masson syndrome
(c) Lennox Gastaut syndrome
(d) West Syndrome

Explanation:

- All the above options are **epileptic syndromes**, among these only **Dyke Davidson Masson syndrome** have characteristic **Childhood Cerebral Hemiatrophy** features.

CAUSES OF CEREBRAL HEMIATROPHY

(A) Congenital

- Idiopathic
- Intrauterine vascular injury

(B) Acquired

- Birth trauma and Congenital malformation
- Perinatal intracranial haemorrhage
- **Rasmussen encephalitis***
- Postictal cerebral hemiatrophy
- Infection – **Herpes Encephalitis, TORCH syndrome, HIV**
- **Vascular/Haematological abnormalities:**
  - ***Dyke Davidson Mason syndrome***
  - **Sturge-Weber syndrome**
- Neoplasia – basal ganglial germinoma
- Radiation and **Phakomatosis** (**Neurofibromatosis**)
- Miscellaneous:
  - Linear Nevus syndrome
  - **Fishman syndrome***
  - **Silver-Russell syndrome***
  - Infantile hemiplegia syndrome
  - Mitochondrial encephalopathy, lactic acidosis, and stroke-like episodes **(MELAS)**

DYKE DAVIDSON MASSON SYNDROME

- **Hemiatrophy or hypoplasia of unilateral cerebral hemisphere** resulting from brain insult in foetal or early childhood period with **compensatory ipsilateral calvarial hypertrophy**
- Insult could be vascular, congenital or acquired ischaemic disease, trauma or inflammation
- In utero gestational vascular occlusion involving middle cerebral vascular territory or coarctation of mid-aortic arch may decrease carotid arterial flow
- Brain growth failure compels inward redirection of nearby calvarial growth accounting for the compensatory calvarial changes like:
  - Enlargement of the frontal sinus
  - Enlargement of frontal sinus
  - Increased width of the diploic space with
  - Elevations of the ipsilateral greater wing of sphenoid and petrous ridge
- MRI features include:

- Unilateral loss of cerebral volume (with or without enlargement of the cortical sulci and cistern).
- Hypoplasia/atrophy of the cerebral peduncle, abnormal myelination and contralateral cerebellar atrophy.
- Capillary malformation.

- Treatment is symptomatic.
- Hemispherectomy: Indications
    - Intractable disabling seizures.
    - Hemiplegia.

Option A: Dravet Syndrome (Severe Myoclonic Epilepsy in Infancy)

- Phenotypic spectrum of **febrile seizure-associated epilepsies.**
- Caused by a de novo mutation, located on **2q24-31 and** encodes for **SCN1A**
- The onset in infancy, characterized by febrile and afebrile unilateral clonic seizures recurring every 1 month.
- Differ from the usual febrile convulsions:
    - Have more prolonged, more frequent, focal and clusters of seizures.
    - Seizures subsequently start to occur with lower fevers and then without fever.
- In 2nd year of life – myoclonus, atypical absences, and partial seizures occur frequently with developmental delay.
- ***Only small patients have abnormality in neuroimaging like – cortical dysplasia, hippocampal sclerosis and focal brain atrophy.***
- Treated with **valproate** and benzodiazepines such as **clobazam or clonazepam.**
- **Lamotrigine**, **carbamazepine**, and **phenytoin** are reported to exacerbate seizures.
- They do not attain remission and have poor prognosis.

Option C: Lennox Gastaut Syndrome

- Starts between the ages of **2-10 years**
- Consists of a triad of:
    - **Developmental delay**
    - **Multiple seizure types** (rule include atypical absences, myoclonic, astatic and tonic seizures.
    - **EEG findings** (1-2 Hz spike–and–slow waves, polyspike bursts in sleep, and a slow background in wakefulness).
- Seizure types that are difficult to control, with long-term cognitive impairment and intractable seizures despite multiple therapies.
- Treatment of seizures varies according to the preponderant seizure type.
    - **For drop attacks** (tonic, atonic, or myoclonic astatic seizures), valproate, lamotrigine, topiramate, clobazam, felbamate, and rufinamide are considered to be effective.
    - For patients who have a preponderance of **atypical absence seizures**, **lamotrigine** or **ethosuximide**.
    - **Clonazepam** is often used as a **rescue medication** for clusters of seizures.
    - In **resistant cases – zonisamide, levetiracetam, acetazolamide, methsuximide, corticosteroids, ketogenic diet, or IVIG** can be used.

Option D: West Syndrome (WS)

- Starts **at 2 and 12 month**

- Consists of a triad of:
  - **Infantile epileptic spasms** (clusters particularly in drowsiness or upon arousal).
  - **Developmental regression.**
  - **Typical EEG** picture called **hypsarrhythmia** (high-voltage, slow, chaotic background with multifocal spikes).
- Idiopathic WS – have normal development before onset.
- Symptomatic WS – have preceding developmental delay owing to perinatal encephalopathies/malformations.
- In boys, WS – caused by *ARX* gene mutations (often associated with ambiguous genitalia and cortical migration abnormalities).
- Treated with **ACTH** (regimen of ACTH (80 mg/mL) is a daily dose of 150 units/m^2 (divided into twice-daily intramuscular injections of 75 units/m^2) administered over a 2-week period with a subsequent gradual taper over a 2-week period.
- Awake and asleep EEGs – done 1, 2 and 4 weeks after the initiation of ACTH to monitor the patient's response.
- **Vigabatrin*** is considered as a drug of second choice.

Ans: (b) Dyke Davidson Masson syndrome

Ref: *Nelson Textbook of Pediatrics, 20th edition, Page 2826 – 2862 and Glob J Health Sci 2013;5(3):195–207*

6. A 15-year-old boy with partial seizure who develops secondary generalization with tonic clonic seizures should be given:

(a) Oxycarbamazepine (b) Zonisamide

(c) Lacosamide (d) Gabapentin

Explanation:

- **Carbamazepine or Oxcarbamazepine** are the drug of choice for **partial seizures** with or **without secondary generalization.**

Choice of Anti Epileptic Drug (AED) according to the seizure type:

No	Seizure type	First line AED	Second line AED
1	Partial onset (with or without secondary generalisation)	OXC, CBZ	PB, CLB
2	Generalised onset tonic clonic	VPA, CBZ, PHT, PB	TPM, LEV
3	Absence	VPA, ESM, LTG	CZP, TPM
4	Myoclonic	VPA, TPM	CZP, LEV
5	Tonic / Atonic	VPA, LTG	CZP, CLB

Choice of AED according to the epileptic syndromes:

No	Epilepsy syndrome	First line AED	Second line AED
1	Juvenile Myoclonic Epilepsy	VPA	PB, CZP
2	Progressive Myoclonic Epilepsy	VPA	CZP
3	Lennox Gastaut Syndrome	VPA, LTG, TPM	CZP, LEV
4	Infantile Spasm	ACTH, VGB	VPA, CLB
5	Benign Rolandic Epilepsy	CBZ, VPA, LTG	PHT, LEV
6	Severe Myoclonic Epilepsy of Infancy	CLB,CZP, VPA	LEV, Stiripentol
7	Landau Kleffner Syndrome	VPA, LTG, STEROIDS	LEV, TPM
8	Myoclonic Astatic Epilepsy	CZP, ZLB, VPZ	LEV, LTG

(PB – Phenobarbitone, PHT – Phenytoin, CBZ – Carbamazepine, VPA – Sodium Valproate, CLB – Clobazam, CZP – Clonazepam, ESM – Ethosuximide, OXC – Oxcarbamazepine, LTG – Lamotrigine, TPM –Topiramate, LEV – Livetiracetam, VGB - Vigabatrin)

Ans: (a) Oxycarbamazepine

Ref: *Seizures and Epilepsy in Children by Prathiba Singhi, Page 111*

7. The first drug of choice for Juvenile myoclonic epilepsy (Janz syndrome):

(a) Oxycarbamazepine (b) Zonisamide

(c) Valproic acid (d) Lacosamide

Explanation:

- **Sodium Valproate** is the first drug of choice in **Juvenile Myoclonic Epilepsy (JME).**

Juvenile Myoclonic Epilepsy (JME):

- Occurs around **puberty** (2:1 female to male ratio).
- Positive family history in 50% of cases.
- **Myoclonic jerks** (within 20 minutes after awakening) with **no loss of consciousness**, mistaken for **post awakening clumsiness**.
- Seizures were precipitated by **sleep deprivation** and **hand activities**.
- **Isolated facial / lingual jerks** precipitated by **talking**.
- Many have **generalized tonic clonic or absence seizures** on **awakening** by 16 years of age.
- **EEG** – Bilateral symmetric diffuse spike waves and poly spike waves which increase with photic stimulation. **Photoparoxysmal response*** is seen.
- ***Valproate*** – Drug of choice and controls seizures in 80% of cases (relapse rate is high on stopping the drug).
- ***Lamotrigine*** preferred in adolescent girls due to risk of Poly Cystic Ovarian Syndrome with valproate.
- ***Azetazolamide*** – Given on long term help in cases with poor response to anti epileptic drugs.

Ans: (c) Valproic acid

Ref: *Seizures and Epilepsy in Children by Prathiba Singhi, Page 98*

8. False about hartnup's disease:

(a) Defect in neutral aminoacid transport (b) Mental retardation is the common presentation

(c) Most children are asymptomatic (d) Photosensitivity

Explanation:

Hartnup Disease

- It is a rare inborn error of metabolism with **autosomal recessive** inheritance.
- Neutral amino acids, including **tryptophan**, are not transported across the brush border epithelium of the intestine and kidneys.
- This results in deficiency of synthesis of **nicotinamide.**
- It causes a **photo-induced pellagra-like syndrome**.
- Increased urinary **monoamine monocarboxylic amino acids**.
- **Cutaneous signs** precede neurologic manifestations.
- Eczematous, occasionally vesiculobullous eruption noted on the face and extremities in a **glove-and-stocking photodistribution**.

- **Hyperpigmentation** and **hyperkeratosis** may supervene and are intensified by further exposure to sunlight.
- Episodic flares may be precipitated by febrile illness, sun exposure, emotional stress, and poor nutrition.
- Emotional instability and **episodic cerebellar ataxia**.
- Neurologic symptoms are fully **reversible**.
- Administration of **nicotinamide** and protection from sunlight improves both cutaneous and neurologic manifestations.

Ans: (b) Mental retardation is the common presentation

Ref: *Nelson's Textbook of Pediatrics, 19th edition*

9. Amount of Protein present in 100 ml of breast milk is:

(a) 2.2 g (b) 1.1 g

(c) 0.55 g (d) 3.3 g

Explanation:

Nutritional values of various milk

Milk source	Quantity	Energy (Kcal)	Protein (g)
Cow	100 ml	67	3.3
Buffalo	100 ml	117	4.3
Goat	100 ml	72	3.7
Human	100 ml	65	1.1

Ans: (b) 1.1 g

Ref: *Vishnu Bhat's Protein Energy Malnutrition, 1st edition, Peepee, Page 51*

DERMATOLOGY

1. Pseudo-isomorphic phenomenon is seen in:

(a) Vitiligo (b) Psoriasis

(c) DLE (d) Plane warts

Explanation:

KOEBNER PHENOMENON

- The **Koebner phenomenon** is the development of **isomorphic** pathologic lesions in the **traumatized uninvolved skin** of patients who have cutaneous diseases.
- Koebner phenomenon signifies activity of the disease.
- **Boyd-Nelder classification of the Koebner phenomenon**

Category I	Psoriasis, lichen planus, vitiligo (true Koebnerization)
Category II	Warts, molluscum contagiosum, pyoderma gangrenosum (pseudo-koebnerization)
Category III	Darier's disease, erythema multiforme, Behcet's disease (occasional lesions), Kaposi's sarcoma, lichen sclerosis
Category IV	Pemphigus vulgaris, eczema, lichen nitidus, dermatitis (poor or questionable herpetiform trauma-induced processes)

TYPES OF KOEBNER PHENOMENON

A. True isomorphic phenomenon:

- Indicates lesions with similar morphology appearing at the sites of trauma
- There appear to be three disease processes that display the true isomorphic response of Koebner:
  - Psoriasis
  - Lichen planus
  - Vitiligo.

B. Pseudoisomorphic phenomenon:

- Characterized by the appearance of morphologically similar skin lesions at the site of injury in lesions
- The Koebner phenomenon also seen in **infectious diseases**
  - **Warts**
  - Molluscum contagiosum
  - Behcet's disease
  - Pyoderma gangrenosum.

C. Occasionally occurring isomorphic phenomenon:

- In this category, diseases occasionally localize to sites of trauma, e.g.:
  - Cancer (gastric, testicular or mammary)
  - Darier's disease
  - Erythema multiforme
  - Hailey-Hailey disease
  - Kaposi's sarcoma

- Kyrle's disease
- Lichen sclerosus et atrophicus
- Pellagra
- Perforating folliculitis
- Reactive perforating collagenosis.

D. **Koebner response in psoriasis:**
- The reported incidence of Koebner response in psoriasis varies from 11-75%.
- The latent period between injury to uninvolved skin and appearance of disease is usually 10-14 days, but it may range from 3 days to several years.

E. **The "reverse" Koebner response:**
- The reverse Koebner reaction is seen when an area of **psoriasis clears** following **injury**, like:
  - Dermabrasion
  - Surgery

F. **Remote reverse Koebner phenomenon**
- It is defined in **vitiligo*** patients, in which **spontaneous repigmentation** is seen in distant patches after autologous **skin graft surgery***.

Ans: (d) Plane warts

Ref: *Madke B, Doshi B, Pande S, Khopkar U. Phenomena in Dermatology, Indian J Dermatol Venereol Leprol 2011;77:264-75*

2. All true regarding spitz nevus except:

(a) Benign tumor
(b) Trunk is the most common site involved
(c) Tumour cells are spindled and epithelioid melanocytes
(d) Treatment is wait and watch

Explanation:

Spitz Naevus

- Melanocytic lesion characterized by **spindled and/or epitheloid naevomelanocytes**.
- The common or classic Spitz naevus is a **benign proliferation** frequently occurring in **children**.
- The **most common sites** for Spitz naevi are the:
  - **Head and neck area** (37%), particularly the face and cheek in children
  - **Lower extremities** (28%) in young adults.
- Due to the very low probability of melanoma in children with typical or classic Spitz naevi, some experts prefer clinical monitoring of these lesions rather than intervention, provided that a close clinical and dermoscopic follow-up is performed.

Ans: (b) Trunk is the most common site involved

Ref: *Rook's Textbook of Dermatology, Page 132.32*

3. Max Joseph Space is a histopatholgoical feature of:

(a) Psoriasis vulgaris
(b) Lichen planus
(c) Pitruasis rosasea
(d) Parapsoriasis

Explanation:

Lichen Planus

- It is a pruritic, inflammatory papulosquamous disorder affecting the skin, mucous membranes, nails and hair follicles.
- **Etiology** – Unknown
  - Genetic predisposition: ***HLA B8***-oral LP; ***HLA-Bw 35***-cutaneous LP
  - Exogenous: ***Primary biliary cirrhosis***, ***alcoholic cirrhosis, hepatitis B, hepatitis C***
  - Drugs cause lichenoid drug eruptions
  - Metals like ***mercury*** (dental amalgams), palladium, gold – oral lichenoid eruptions
- **Clinical Features:**
  - 30-60 years; children–4% of cases, childhood LP more common in India
  - ***Skin***
    - Intensely **pruritic, flat topped**, shiny, polygonal, violaceous papules and plaques
    - Predominantly **flexor distribution** – flexor of wrist, forearm, legs, trunk, glans penis (cf–psoriasis another papulosquamous disorder has predominant extensor distribution)
    - ***Wickham's striae****–network of greyish white streaks on papules seen on pressing with glass slide after application of oil – corresponds to wedge shaped hypergranulosis seen on histopathology
    - ***Koebner/isomorphic phenomenon**** common
    - Annular LP–glans penis
    - Hypertrophic LP–shins
    - Actinic LP–sun exposed areas
  - ***Oral:***
    - Classical type is reticulate pattern–***white/violaceous lacy reticular network*** of coalesent papules in buccal mucosa and tongue; usually asymptomatic
    - Most common pattern – ***ulcerative/erosive LP***
  - ***Nail:***
    - 5-10% cases
    - **Thinning of nail plate** (cf psoriasis – thickening of nail plate), longitudinal ridging, roughening of nail plate (***trachyonychia****) and nail dystrophy involving all 20 nails called 20 nail dystrophy (also seen in alopecia areata)
    - Classical/characteristic nail finding (but not common finding)–***pterygium* formation*** (proximal nail fold fuses with nail bed)
  - ***Hair follicles: Lichen Planopilaris – scarring alopecia*.***
- **Histopathology:**
  - Hyperkeratosis
  - Wedge shaped hypergranulosis (psoriasis – hypogranulosis)
  - Irregular acanthosis (psoriasis – regular acanthosis)
  - ***Saw tooth rete ridges**** (psoriasis – elephant foot/camel foot like/club shaped rete ridges)
  - Basal layer vacuolar degeneration
  - Band like dermal lymphocytic infiltrate hugging epidermis
  - ***Max Joseph spaces**** – subepidermal clear zone (subepidermal clear zone in lepromatous leprosy is called Grenz zone)
  - Melanin incontinence

- **Treatment** – Steroids (topical/intralesionsal/systemic), retinoids, cyclosporine, PUVA photochemotherapy, dapsone, methotrexate

ALSO NOTE:

Lichen Planus–"8 P's"

- **P**apulosquamous disorder
- **P**ruritic
- **P**lane topped
- **P**olygonal/**p**olyangular
- **P**urple coloured
- **P**apules
- **P**laques
- **P**igmentation after healing
- **P**terygium formation in nails

Ans: (b) Lichen planus

Ref: *Rook's Textbook of Dermatology, Page 431*

4. True statement regarding molluscum contagiosum:

(a) Associated more severe in atopic dermatitis
(b) Can be treated by cantharidin
(c) Self-limiting even in HIV
(d) Caused by Flavivirus

Explanation:

MOLLUSCUM CONTAGIOSUM

- Skin infection caused by the **Pox virus, Molluscum contagiosum** virus.
- The individual lesion is a **shiny, pearly white, hemispherical, umbilicated** papule which may show a central pore.
- Widespread and **refractory mollusca** on the **face** are seen most commonly in **HIV disease** and also with **iatrogenic immunosuppression**.

TREATMENT

First Line

- **Caustic destruction:** Cantharidin, trichloroacetic acid, diluted liquefied phenol.
- **Irritant:** Salicylic acid, adapalene, nitric oxide cream, potassium hydroxide, benzoyl peroxide, lemon myrtle oil, tea tree oil.
- Surgical irritation.

Second Line

- **Immunological:** Diphencyprone, imiquimod, interferon, cimetidine, intralesional immunotherapy.
- Surgical removal.

Third Line

- Cidofovir
- Paclitaxel

Ans: (b) Can be treated by cantharidin

Ref: *Rook's Textbook of Dermatology, Page 25.14*

5. Keratoderma blenorrhagica is found in:

(a) Reiter's syndrome
(b) Psoriasis
(c) Lichen planus
(d) Behcet's syndrome

Explanation:

Keratoderma Blennorrhagicum (also known as Keratoderma Blennorrhagica)

- These lesions are seen in **reactive arthritis** (in 15% of male patients).
- Found on the ***palms and soles*** but which may spread to the ***scrotum, scalp and trunk***.
- The appearance is usually of a ***vesico-pustular waxy lesion*** with a yellow brown colour.
- These lesions may join together to form larger crusty plaques with desquamating edges.
- ***Resemble psoriasis*** in morphology and distribution.

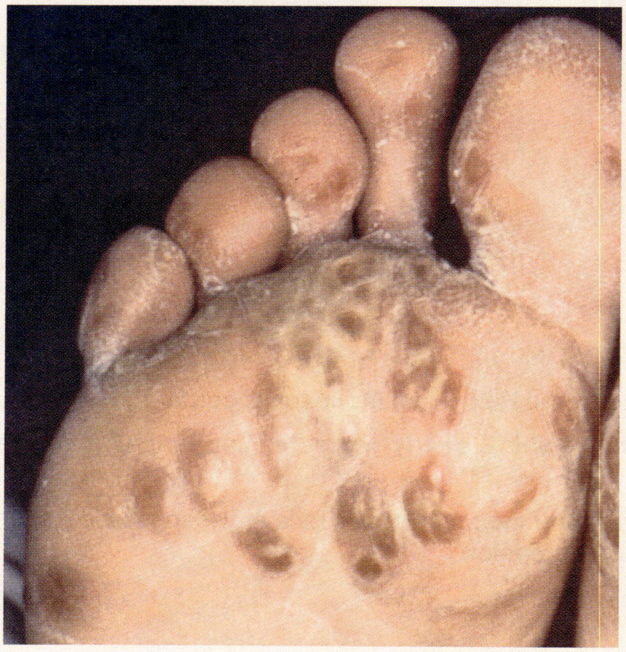

Figure: Keratoderma blennorrhagicum

REITER'S SYNDROME

Triad of Symptoms:

- Inflammatory arthritis of **large joints**
- Inflammation of the **eyes** in the form of **conjunctivitis or uveitis**
- **Urethritis** in men or **cervicitis** in women.
    - Simply, Triad of **urethritis, arthritis and conjunctivitis***
- **Cutaneous eruption:**
    - Limpet like scales
    - ***Circinate balanitis***

- Shallow painless ulcers of palate, tongue and glans
- ***Keratoderma blennorrhagica*** – palms and soles

- **Enthesitis** involving **Achilles tendon** causing heel pain
- **RF–seronegative**
- **HLA B 27** in 80% of cases
- Prior episode of urogenital or gastrointestinal infection

Intestinal infections

- Salmonella
- Shigella
- Campylobacter

Sexually transmitted infections

- Chlamydia trachomatis
- Ureaplasma urealyticum
- Neisseria gonorrheae

- **Treatment**: Methotrexate

Ans: (a) Reiter's syndrome

Ref: *Essentials in Dermatology, 2nd edition*

6. True regarding keratoacanthoma:

(a) Central necrosis is uncommon
(b) Known as molluscum sebaceum
(c) Caused by pox virus
(d) Heals without scarring

Explanation:

KERATOACANTHOMA

- **Also known as Molluscum sebaceum**
- Rapidly growing tumor
- Developing on **sun-exposed skin**
- **Potential to regress**
- Classification is controversial
- Probable variant of **squamous cell carcinoma**

RISK FACTORS

- Most commonly in older **males > 50 years**
- **Sun-exposed** skin
- Similar risk factors to **squamous cell carcinoma**
- Variants with **multiple lesions**
- ***Fergusson-Smith syndrome***
  - Autosomal **dominant**
  - **Scottish** ancestry
  - More common in **men**

- **Younger** patients
- **Multiple lesions** (100s) sun-exposed and sun-protected sites
- Lower likelihood of **involution**

- ***Grzybowski syndrome***
  - No gender predilection
  - Multiple **eruptive lesions** (100s to 1000s)
  - **Sun-exposed** sites or generalized
  - May involve **mucous membranes**
- ***Muir-Torre syndrome***

Pathology

- Symmetrical, cup-shaped, endo-/exophytic tumor with collarette and central keratin plug
- Well-differentiated squamous epithelium with glassy, pale cytoplasm
- **Mitotic activity** low and generally basal
- **Neutrophilic microabscesses** in tumor epithelium may be present
- Entrapped **elastic fibers in center of lesion** sometimes evident
- Regressing lesions demonstrate flattening of epithelium, loss of keratin plug; dermal, foreign-body, giant cell reaction often present
- **Central necrosis** is **common**

Presentation

- Solitary or multiple lesions; solitary more common
- Cup-shaped, rapidly growing lesion on sun-exposed site
- Keratin core with raised, erythematous border
- **1 to 2 cm** in diameter
- Giant keratoacanthoma: **>3 cm** diameter
- Involutes over several weeks, **leaving scar**
- Typical lesion life cycle is **5 to 6 months**

Prognosis and Treatment

- Overall **good prognosis**
- Potential to **regress** without treatment
- **Rare lesions** reported to **metastasize**
- **Treatment**:
  - Surgical **excision**
  - Intralesional **methotrexate**
  - Systemic **retinoids** in patients with multiple lesions

Ans: (b) Known as molluscum sebaceum

Ref: *Brinster NK, Dermatopathology: High-Yield Pathology, Page 380-381*

ANESTHESIOLOGY

1. Examine the CT Abdomen image of a patient posted for surgery. Which drug should not be given intra operatively in this condition?

(a) IV Atropine

(b) IV Esmolol

(c) IV Phoxybenxamine/Phentolamine

(d) IV Normal saline

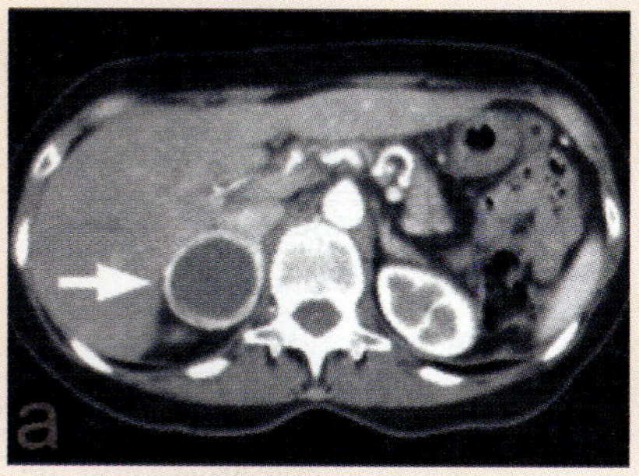

Explanation:

CT image is showing **suprarenal mass** arising from adrenal gland, probably a **pheochromocytoma**

PHEOCHROMOCYTOMA

- **Catecholamine**-secreting tumors of **chromaffin tissue.**
- Usually located in the **adrenal medulla or sympathetic paraganglia**, but may be found anywhere chromaffin tissue exists.
- **90%** are found in the **adrenal medulla.**
- The catecholamines are **epinephrine, norepinephrine and dopamine**. These three compounds are found in the chromaffin cells of the sympathetic nervous system, which includes the adrenal medulla, aberrant tissue along the sympathetic chain and paraganglia.
- The **classic triad is:**
  - Severe headache
  - Diaphoresis
  - Palpitations.
- Pheochromocytomas occur in **both sexes** with peak incidence in the **third to fifth decades** of life.
- Approximately 5% of cases of pheochromocytomas are inherited as an **autosomal dominant trait** either alone or as part of the neoplastic syndrome, multiple endocrine adenomatosis.

Multiple Endocrine Adenomatosis	
Type IIa (Sipple syndrome)	Parathyroid adenoma/hyperplasia Medullary carcinoma of thyroid Pheochromocytoma
Type IIb	Medullary carcinoma of the thyroid Mucosal adenomas Marfanoid appearance Pheochromocytoma
von Hippel-Lindau syndrome	Hemangioblastoma of the retina, cerebellum, or other parts of the CNS, pheochromocytoma
Neurofibromatosis	Neurofibromas, café-au-lait spots, axillary or inguinal freckling, optic nerve glioma, pheochromocytoma

Lab Investigation for Pheochromocytoma:

Diagnostic Test	Normal Values	Pheochromocytoma
Blood		
Plasma catecholamines	<1,000 pg/mL	> 2000 pg/mL
Urine (24 hours collection)		
Catecholamines	<125 μg	>1,200 μg
Norepinephrine	<100 μg	Increased
Epinephrine	<1 μg	Increased
Metanephrines	<1.6 mg	> 2.5 mg
Vanilylmandelic acid	<8 mg	> 10 mg
Confirmation if test results are equivocal		
Clonidine suppression of norepinephrine secretion	Suppressed in essential hypertensive patients	Not suppressed
Localization of tumor		
Magnetic resonance imaging		
Computed tomography		
Scintigraphy with metainodobenzyl guanidine (MIBG)		
Selective adrenal venous catheterization and sampling		

- **Drugs to be avoided:**
  - **Atropine**
  - **Pancuronium**
  - Ketamine
  - Ephedrine
  - **Morphine**
  - Curare
  - **Atracurium**
  - **Pancuronium**
  - Droperidril
  - **Halothane**
  - Metaclopromide
  - Cocaine
- **Drugs used to control Hypretension:**
  - **Phentolamine (DOC)**
  - Diltiazem
  - **Esmolol**
  - Hydralazine
  - Labetalol
  - Propanolol
  - $MGSO_4$
  - Nitroprusside

- Nicardepine
- Lidocaine (to control arrhythmias)

Ans: (a) IV Atropine

Ref: *Stoelting's Anesthesia Coexisting Disease, 7th edition*

2. Regarding Morphine and Tramadol, which statement is true?

(a) Morphine is less potent than tramadol
(b) Tramadol exhibits NMDA receptor antagonism
(c) Pruritus is a common side effect of tramadol
(d) Tramadol is a synthetic codeine derivative

Explanation:

Tramadol:

- Is a **centrally acting** synthetic **opioid** (**codeine derivative).**
- 5 times less potent than Morphine.
- Analgesic effect due to:
  - Affinity for **mu, kappa and delta** opoid receptor.
  - Enhances the function of spinal descending inhibitory pathway by inhibition of the neuraonal uptake of Norepinephrine and 5-hydroxytryptamine (Serotonin).
- Is a racemic mixture of 2 enantiomers.
- Produce analgesia with absence of depression of ventilation, less tolerance, dependence and abuse potential.
- **Use:**
  - Can administer orally, IM, IV for **analgesia** and also as adjuvant in **regional analgesia**
  - Treatment of **postoperative shivering**
  - Treatment of **chronic cancer pain**.
- **Disadvantages:**
  - Drug related seizures (avoid in patients with epilepsy).
  - Interaction with caumadine (warfarin) anticoagulants.

Comparison of Opioid Drugs

Opioid	Natural/ synthetic	PPB (%)	CSH (Min)	Active Metabolite	Potency in Compare to Morphine
Morphine	Natural	35	–	Morphine 6 glucoronide	1
Heroin	Synthetic	30	–		–
Meperidine	Synthetic	70	–	Normeperidine	1/10
Fentanyl	Synthetic	84	260	Norfentanyl	75-125 times
Sufentanyl	Synthetic	93	30	Desmethylsufentanyl	12 times of fentanyl
Alfentanyl	Synthetic	92	60	Noralfentanyl	1/10 of fentanyl
Remifentanyl	Synthetic	66-93	4	–	5-10 times of fentanyl
Tramadol	Synthetic	50	–	O-desmethyltramadol	5 times less than Morphine

- PPB–plasma protein binding
- CST–context sensitive half life

Ans: (d) Tramadol is a synthetic codeine derivative

Ref: *Stoelting's Pharmacology and Physiology in Anesthtic Practice, 6th edition*

3. Which of the following is the most common initial manifestation of malignant hyperthermia?

(a) Hyperkalemia
(b) Increased distal esophageal temperature
(c) Increased PET CO_2
(d) Red discoloration of urine

Explanation:

MALIGNANT HYPERTHERMIA (MH)

- Rare genetic disease (1:15,000 in pediatric patients and 1:40,000 adult patients) characterized by an **acute hypermetabolic state** within muscle tissue **following induction of general anesthesia**.
- **Risk Factors:**
  - Drugs:
    - **Halogenated general anesthetics** (**Ether**, **cyclopropane**, **halothane***, **isoflurane**, **sevoflurane**, **desflurane**, enflurane, methoxyflurane).
    - Nondepolarizing muscle relaxants – **Succinylcholine***.
  - Family history of Malignant hyperthermia.
  - **Myopathy**
- **Pathology:**
  - The initial focus of investigations was on an abnormal **ryanodine Ryr1 receptor** in patients with MH.
  - This **calcium channel receptor** is responsible for **calcium release** from the **sarcoplasmic reticulum** and plays a critical role in **muscle depolarization**.
  - However, further studies have revealed that many MH patients have a **normal ryanodine receptor** and that abnormalities in **secondary messengers and modulators of calcium release**, such as **fatty acids** and **phosphatidylinositol**, may be present.
  - An abnormal **sodium channel** in **skeletal muscle** may also play a role in some patients.
- **Sign and symptoms:**

Hypermetabolism	Increased sympathetic activity	Muscle damage	Hyperthermia
• ET CO_2 production • Increase O_2 consumption • Decreases mixed venous O_2 tension • Cyanosis • Mottling	• Tachycardia • Hypertension • Arrhythmia	• Masseter spasm • Generalized rigidity • ↑Serum creatinine kinase • ↑K • ↑Na • ↑PO_4 • Mayoglobinuria	• Fever • Shivering

- **Treatment**–Malignant Hyperthermia Protocol
  - Discontinue volatile anesthetic and succinylcholine. Call for help.
  - **Hyperventilate** with 100% O_2 at high flows.
  - Administer **sodium bicarbonate**, 1–2 mEq/kg intravenously.
  - Mix **dantrolene sodium** with sterile distilled water and administer 2.5 mg/kg intravenously as soon as possible.
  - Institute cooling measures (lavage, cooling blanket, cold intravenous solutions).

- Administer **inotropes** and **antiarrhythmic agents** as necessary.
- Administer additional doses of **dantrolene** if needed.
- Change anesthetic tubing and soda lime.
- Monitor urinary output, K+, Ca2+, blood gases, end-tidal carbon dioxide; perform clotting studies.
- **Treat severe hyperkalemia** with dextrose, 25–50 g intravenously, and regular insulin, 10–20 U intravenously (adult dose).
- Consider invasive monitoring of arterial blood pressure and central venous pressure.

ALSO NOTE:

What does $PetCO_2$ mean?

- **Quantitative waveform capnography** is the continuous, noninvasive measurement and graphical display of **end-tidal carbon dioxide/$ETCO_2$** (also called **$PetCO_2$**). Capnography uses a sample chamber/sensor placed for optimum evaluation of expired CO_2.

Ans: (c) Increased $PETCO_2$

Ref: *Stoelting's Pharmacology and Physiology in Anesthetic Practice, 6th edition*

4. The patient with LEAST risk of pulmonary aspiration of gastric contents during induction of anesthesia is:

(a) Markedly obese and NPO for eight hours

(b) Fed coffee four hours before elective surgery

(c) Scheduled for elective cesarean delivery and NPO for 20 hours

(d) NPO for four hours after a full meal

Explanation:

NPO Guidelines:

Ingested material	Minimum fasting period before surgery (in hours)
Clear fluid	2
Breast milk	4
Formula feed	6
Non-humam milk	6
Light meal	6
Fried heavy meal	8

Risk of aspiration increases in:

- Emergency surgery*
- Inadequate airway protection
- **Abdominal pathology***
- **Obesity***
- Opioid medication
- **Neurologic deficit***
- **Lithotomy**

- Difficult intubation
- **Reflux**
- Hiatal hernia
- **Pregnancy***

Ans: (d) NPO for four hours after a full meal

Ref: *Clinical Anaesthesia Barash, 8th edition*

5. Which of the following Mapleson systems has no rebreathing bag?

(a) A (b) C

(c) D (d) E

Explanation:

- The breathing system (breathing or patient circuit, respiratory circuit or system) is a gas pathway connected to the patient, through which gas flows occur at respiratory pressures, and into which a controlled composition of a gas mixture is dispensed.
- The Mapleson systems are characterized by the absence of unidirectional valves to direct gases to or from the patient.
    - Because there is no device for absorbing CO_2, the fresh gas flow must wash CO_2 out of the circuit.
    - For this reason, these systems are sometimes called *carbon dioxide washout circuits* or *flow-controlled breathing systems* or Open circuit.
- The **Mapleson system's** components include:
    - A reservoir bag
    - Corrugated tubing
    - APL valve
    - Fresh gas inlet; and
    - Patient connection.
- **Mapleson A Circuit:**
    - Is also called **Magill circuit**
    - Used for spontaneous ventilation
- **Mapleson D Circuit:**
    - Is also called **Bain's circuit**
    - Used for controlled ventilation
- **Mapleson E circuit:**
    - Is called as **Ayer's T-piece**
    - Used in pediatric control ventilation
- **Mapleson F circuit:**
    - Is called **Jackson reis modification** (placement of reservoir bag)
    - Used in pediatric control ventilation.

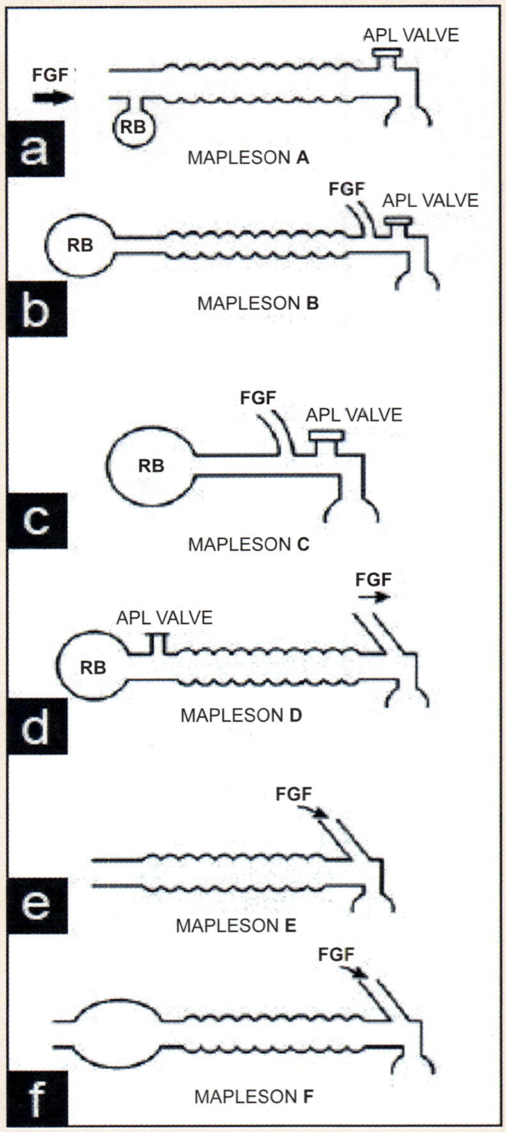

Ans: (d) E

Ref: *Dorsch and Dorsch's Understanding of Anesthesia Equipments, 8th edition*

6. Which of the following induction agent causes least respiratory depression?

(a) Midazolam (b) Ketamine

(c) Propofol (d) Thiopentone

Explanation:

	Anaesthetic agents	Thiopenthol sodium	Propofol	Ketamine	Midazolam	Etomidate
Pharma-cokinetics	MOA	GABA receptor agonist	GABA recepter agonist	NMDA antagonist	GABA receptor agonist	GABA receptor agonist
	Metabolism	Liver by hydroxylation	Liver by conjugation	Liver by demethylation-active metabolite nor ketamine	Liver by hydroxylation	Liver by ester hydrolysis
	Excretion	Renal	Renal and lung	Renal	Renal	Renal
	PPB in %	80	75	70	98	75
	pH	11	4.4	7.5	6.15	6.9
	T1/2 (min)	8-10	10	2 hours	2 hours	30
	Onset of action	One arm circulation time	1 min	1 min	One arm circulation time	One arm circulation time
	Duration of action	12 hours	24 hours	3 hours	4 hours	6 hours
Pharma-codynamics	CNS	↓ ICT, $CMRO_2$, CBF	↓ ICT, $CMRO_2$, CBF	↑ICT, $CMRO_2$, CBF	↓ ICT, $CMRO_2$, CBF	↓ ICT, $CMRO_2$,CBF
	CVS	↑ HR ↓MAP	no change-HR ↓MAP	↑↑HR, ↑↑ BP	↑ HR ↓MAP	↑ HR ↓MAP
	RS	↓ RR, Broncho-constriction	↓ RR, Bronchoconstriction	- RR, Brocho dilation	↓ RR,	↓ RR, Bronchoconstriction
	Renal	↓RBF	↓RBF	↑RBF	↓RBF	↓RBF
	Hepatic	↓HBF	↓HBF	↑HBF	↓HBF	↓HBF
Indication		• Induction of anesthesia • Status epilepticus	• Induction of Anesthesia • TIVA • ICU sedation • Agent of choice for day care surgery	• Induction of anesthesia in asthmatic patients and shock • Neuroleptic anesthesia • Refractory bronchospasm	• Anxiolytic • TIVA • Induction of anesthesia • Sedation	• Induction agent of choice in patient with and shock, trauma and cardiac disease
Contraindication		1. Acute intermittent porphyria 2. Sulpha drug allergy	1. Hypotension and Shock 2. Egg allergy	1. ↑ ICT 2. CAD 3. HTN 4. Acute glaucoma 5. ICSOL 6. Bleeding diathesis	1. Hypotension	Non specific
Specific adverse effects		1. Anaphylatic reaction 2. Intraarterial injection causes gangrene of finger	1. Pain on injection 2. Thrombophlebitis 3. Propofol infusion syndrome 4. Abuse potential	1. Emergency delirium 2. ↑ all pressures 3. Bleeding by inhibition platelet aggregation	1. Respiratory depression and hypotension	1. Adrenocortical suppression 2. Myoclonic movements

Ans: (b) Ketamine

Ref: *Stoelting's Pharmacology and Physiology in Anesthetic Practice, 6th edition*

7. Drug producing haematological side effect is:

(a) Nitrous oxide
(b) Halothane
(c) Ketamine
(d) Sevoflurane

Explanation:

Nitrous oxide *produces* ***Aplastic anemia*** **and** ***Megaloblastic anemia***

NITROUS OXIDE (LAUGHING GAS)

- Stored as liquid in ***blue*** color cylinder
- **1.5** times more heavier than ***air***
- **35** times more soluble than ***nitrogen***

Anesthetic Properties

- It is not a complete anesthetic
- It is used as a ***carrier gas*** to other anesthetics
- MAC is ***104%*** (It is not possible to deliver, so not a complete anesthetic)
- Maximum concentration which can be given is ***66%***
- A minimum of 33% of Oxygen has to be given (Otherwise can cause severe hypoxia)
- It is usually given as N_2O 66% and O_2 33% mixture
- Blood gas coefficient is ***0.47*** making it agent with faster induction and recovery
- ***Good analgesic***
- ***Not a muscle relaxant***
- When given with other inhalational agent, it increases the concentration of that agent ***(Second gas effect)*** and also its own concentration (***Concentration effect***)
- Sudden stoppage can lead to ***Diffusion Hypoxia*** (Should always be tapered slowly by giving 100% oxygen)

Metabolism

- It is ***not metabolized*** in human body
- It is excreted unchanged in lungs
- Small amount is excreted via skin (Percutaneous excretion)
- Impurities in N_2O cylinder can cause severe laryngospasm, methemoglobinemia and Pulmonary edema

Systemic Actions

- **CVS:** It does not depress the myocardium in vivo, so it can be safely used in patients with cardiac disease and shock
- **CNS:** It increases cerebral metabolic rate and raises intracranial tension
- **RS:** It causes tachypnea and decrease tidal volume, maintaining minute volume
- Ventilatory response to hypoxia is blunted
- No significant effect on Liver and Kidneys

Side Effects

- **Hematological:** It inactivates vitamin B_{12} (If used for >6 hours) → defective folate metabolism → Bone marrow depression → ***Aplastic anemia*** and ***Megaloblastic anemia.***
- **CNS:** Vitamin B_{12} deficiency can cause Demyelination of spinal cord (Subacute degeneration of spinal cord) especially involving posterior columns and lateral spinothalamic tracts.
- **Closed Gas Spaces:** Compliant spaces like gut, penumoperitoneum, pneumothorax and non-compliant spaces like middle ear cavity, pneumoencephalum can develop very high pressure following nitrous oxide inhalation.
- This happens because for 1 mole of nitrogen removed, 35 moles of nitrous oxide enter (35 times more soluble than nitrogen.
- Therefore, Nitrous oxide is **contraindicated** in:
  - Pneumothorax
  - Pneumoperitoneum
  - Pneumoencephalum
  - Middle ear surgery
  - Posterior fossa surgery
  - Laproscopic surgery
  - Acute intestinal obstruction and volvulus of gut
  - Eye surgeries

Uses in Anesthesia

- As a supplement to anesthesia (not a complete anesthetic)
- As a carrier gas for inhalational agents
- As analgesic in obstetrics, dental pain, burn dressing and acute trauma

Ans: (a) Nitrous oxide

Ref: *Ajay Yadav, Short Textbook of Anesthesia, 2nd edition, Page 69*

8. In spinal anaesthesia, drug is injected between:

(a) Between pia and arachnoid
(b) Between dura and arachnoid
(c) Between pia and dura
(d) Outside dura

Explanation:

SUBARACHNOID SPACE (Spinal Anesthesia)

- Cerebrospinal fluid is found in the spinal space between the **pia and arachnoid** (**subarachnoid space**).

EPIDURAL SPACE (Epidural anesthesia)

- The epidural space is a potential space.
- It contains connective tissue, venous plexuses and adipose tissue.
- It is found between the connective tissue covering the vertebrae and the **ligamentum flavum** posteriorly and the **dura mater** anteriorly.
- Laterally it is bound by the **pedicles** and the **intervertebral foramina**.
- It extends from the **foramen magnum**, where the dura is fused to the base of the skull, to the **sacral hiatus**.

- The plica mediana dorsalis is a connective tissue band that may extend from the dura mater to the ligamentum flavum, which divides the posterior epidural space into right and left compartments.
- Clinically, this is significant because it may affect the spread of epidurally injected medications.

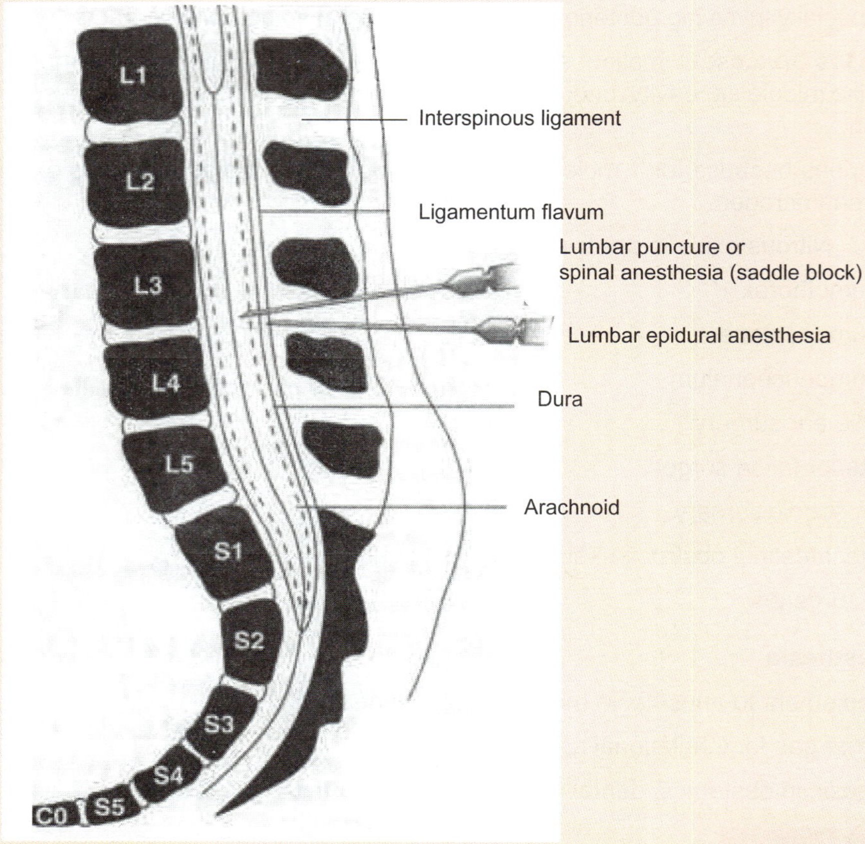

Ans: (a) Between pia and arachnoid

Ref: *Miller Textbook of Anaesthesia, 6th edition*

RADIOLOGY AND RADIOTHERAPY

1. Hot cross bun sign on MRI is seen in:

(a) Unverricht-Lundborg disease
(b) Multisystem atrophy
(c) Huntington disease
(d) Hereditary spastic paraplegia

Explanation:

- Hot cross bun sign refers to the **cruciform-shaped hyperintensity on T2W axial magnetic resonance images (MRI)** in **multisystem atrophy** due to the selective loss of **myelinated transverse pontocerebellar fibers** and neurons in the **pontine raphe** and **sparing** of the **pontine tegmentum and corticospinal tracts**.

Multisystem Atrophy (MSA)

- Sporadic progressive neurodegenerative disorder of adult onset, involving the **basal ganglia** and the **olivopontocerebellar complex** to varying degrees.
- It commonly presents with **Parkinsonian symptoms** and **cerebellar ataxia** and depending on which of these symptoms predominates, is classified as:
  - **MSA-Parkinsonian predominant (MSA-P);** and
  - MSA-Cerebellar predominant (MSA-C) respectively.
- **Hot cross bun sign*** is a manifestation of **pontine atrophy** in MSA and is more commonly found in MSA-C. **Infratentorial atrophy** with hyperintense signal in the **middle cerebral peduncle** and the hot cross bun sign in the pons can provide helpful adjunct in making the diagnosis of MSA.

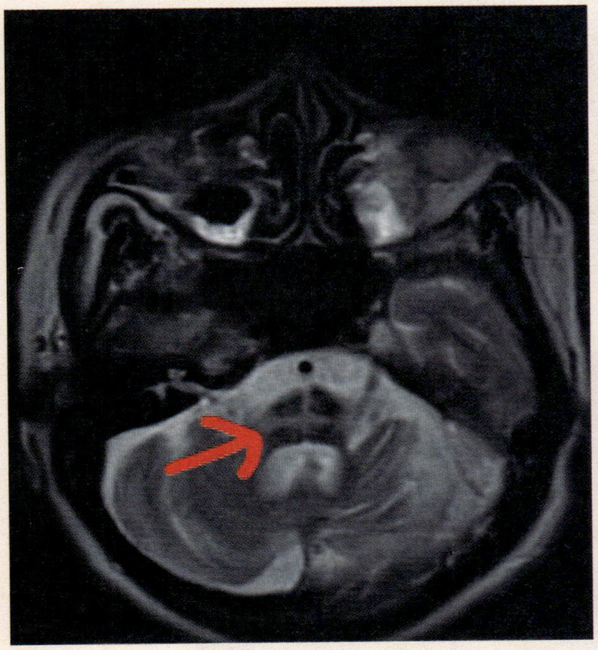

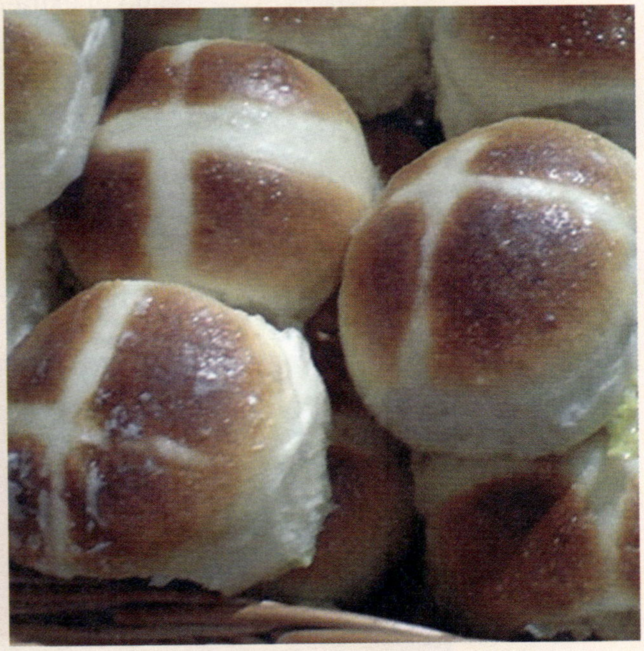

Ans: (b) Multisystem atrophy

Ref: *Neurol India, 2009 Jan-Feb;57(1):104-5*

2. **Examine the given CT Brain picture. What is the most probable diagnosis?**
   (a) Ependymoma
   (b) Meningioma
   (c) Glioblastoma
   (d) Hemangioblastoma

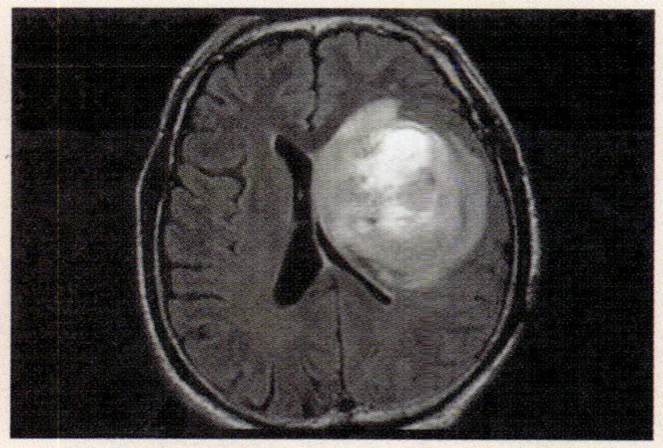

Explanation:

- Axial FLAIR MR Image of the Brain shows a large ill-defined T2 heterogeneously **hyperintense** lesion in the **left temporofrontal lobe** with **peripheral hyperintense vasogenic edema**, with **mid line shift** and **mass effect** on the **ipsilateral lateral ventricle**.
- Rapidly enlarging malignant **astrocytic tumor** (**Glioblastoma**) characterized by **necrosis and neovascularity**
- Most common of all primary intracranial neoplasms.
- Best diagnostic clue: Thick, irregular-enhancing rind of neoplastic tissue surrounding necrot c core.
- Location: **Supratentorial** white matter **most common.**

Other Options:

- **Ependymoma**: Intraventricular tumor.
- **Hemangioblastoma**: Infratentorial, cystic with mural nodule.
- **Meningioma:** Extra axial lesion.

Sign of extra-axial location

Definitive sign	Suggestive sign
• **CSF** cleft between brain and lesion	• Peripheral, broadly base along calvarium
• **Vessels** interposed between brain and lesion	• Overlying bone change
• **Cortex** between brain and lesion	• Enhancement of adjacent meninges
• **Dura** (Meninges) between brain and lesion	• Displacement of brain from the skull

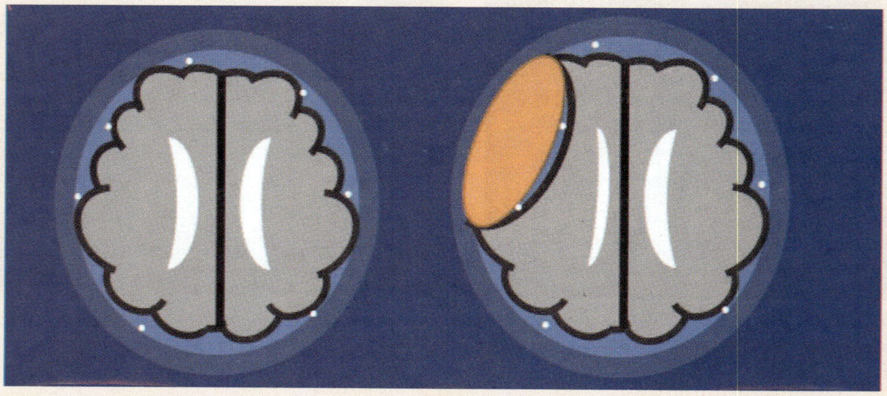

Ans: (c) Glioblastoma

Ref: *Diagnostic Imaging Brain by Anne G.Osborn, Page 1620*

3. True statement regarding nitrates in myocardial perfusion study:

(a) Stress agent

(b) Decreased myocardial flow in ischemia

(c) Enhances the detection of myocardial viability in Thallium 201 radiopharmaceutical agent

(d) Reduced collateral flow into ischemic zone

Explanation:

- Use of **thrombolysis** and **aspirin** has reduced mortality, but **reperfusion** may produce **myocardial salvage**, and if a partially infarcted region supplied by a stenotic artery remains, this may present a greater risk of future ischemic events.
- Use of **treadmill exercise ECG** for **risk stratification** after thrombolysis for myocardial infarction has been shown to be **poorly predictive of future cardiac risk**.
- **^{201}Tl imaging** has been widely used for **risk stratification** after acute myocardial infarction. It has been demonstrated to be **superior** to either **exercise ECG or coronary arteriography** at predicting high- and low-risk groups.
- **Nitrate** is known to enhance the relative flow to severely ischemic segments because of vasodilatation of the stenotic artery and thus improve ^{201}Tl delivery.
- Nitrates may also increase flow to peri-infarct regions by enhancing collateral flow distal to an occluded coronary artery.

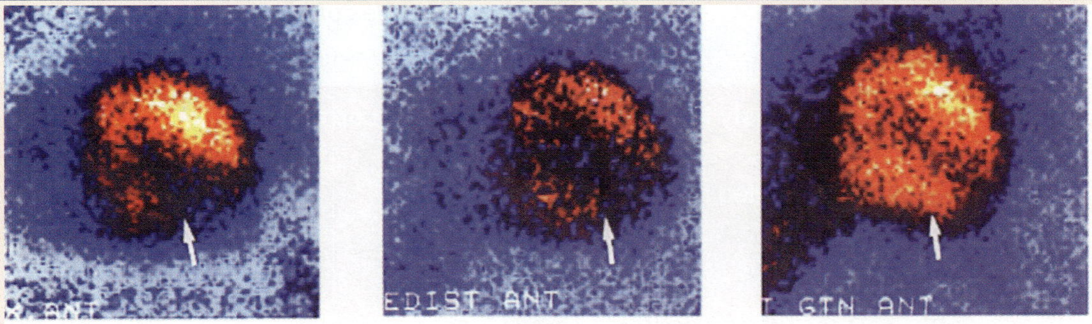

Exercise (left), redistribution (center), and nitrate (NTG)-enhanced rest ^{201}Tl images (right) in anterior projection of a patient with inferior myocardial infarction.

**Inferior wall defect (arrows) shows no reversibility on redistribution imaging but almost complete normalization by nitrate-enhanced rest imaging.

Ans: (c) Enhances the detection of myocardial viability in Thallium 201 radiopharmaceutical agent

Ref: *Circulation 1997;96:2932-2937*

4. The order of imaging methods (from worst to best) with respect to visibility of detail (resolution) is:

(a) Gamma camera, fluoroscopy, CT

(b) Ultrasound, fluoroscopy, radiography

(c) Gamma camera, fluoroscopy, MRI

(d) Radiography, fluoroscopy, MRI

Explanation:

- The order of imaging methods (from worst to best) with respect to visibility of detail (resolution) is **Gamma camera → Ultrasound → MRI → CT → Fluorosocpy → Radiography***.

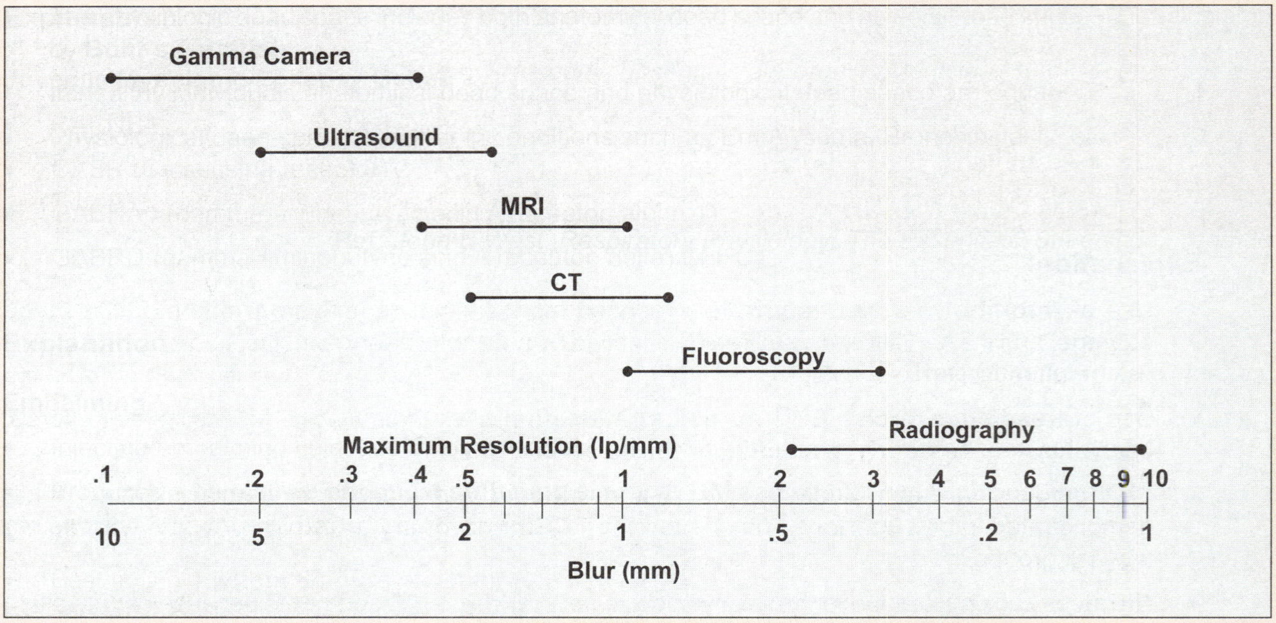

Comparison of Blur and Resolution Values for Different Imaging Methods

Ans: (d) Radiography, fluoroscopy, MRI

Ref: *Physical Principles of Medical Imaging, 2nd edition, Page 7*

5. Eye-of-the-tiger sign is previously known to have one-to-one correlation with which of the following conditions?

(a) Pantothenate kinase-associated neurodegeneration (PKAN)

(b) Neurofibromatosis Type-1

(c) Glomus tumor

(d) Alobar Holoprosencephaly

Explanation:

- **Eye-of-the-tiger sign** represents marked low signal intensity of the globus palladi on T2W MRI images.
- This low signal surrounds a central, small hyperintense area, producing the eye-of-the-tiger appearance.
- The sign is seen in what was once known as **Hallervorden-Spatz (HS) syndrome** but is now called **neurodegeneration** with brain iron accumulation (**NBIA**) or **pantothenate kinase II (PANC2)-associated neurodegeneration.**
- The marked low signal intensity of the **globus palladi** is a result of excessive **iron accumulation** and the central high signal is attributed to **gliosis**, increased **water content**, and **neuronal loss with disintegration**, **vacuolization**, and **cavitation of the neuropil**.
- The sign can be seen in other **extrapyramidal Parkinsonian disorders** such as:
  - Cortical-basal ganglionic degeneration
  - Steele-Richardson-Olszewski syndrome
  - Early-onset levodopa-responsive Parkinsonism
  - Wilson disease
  - Organophosphate poisoning
  - Normal finding on a 3T magnet.

Other Options

- **Neurofibromatosis Type-I – Bare Orbit Sign***
- **Glomus Tumor – Salt and Pepper Sign***
- **Alobar Holoprosencephaly – Pancake Brain Sign***

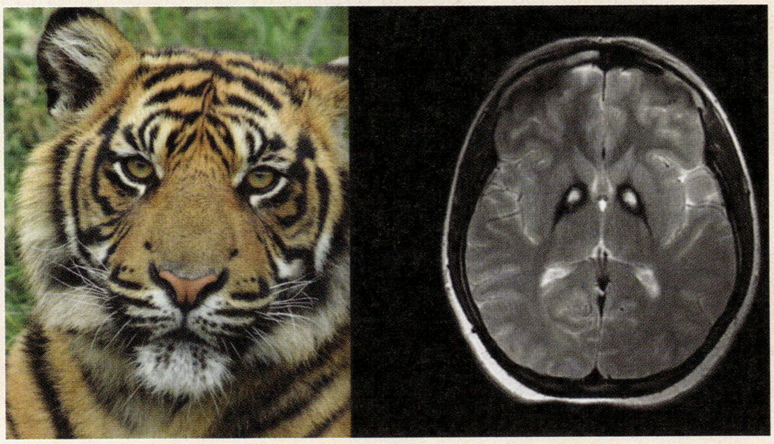

Axial T2W MRI image of the brain shows hypointensity of the globus palladi (arrows). There is relative hyperintensity of the central part, giving the globus palladi the appearance of the eyes of a tiger.

Ans: (a) Pantothenate kinase-associated neurodegeneration (PKAN)

Ref: *Indian J Radiol Imaging 2009 May;19(2), Page 135-145*

6. Best Advantage of doing Transcranial Doppler Ultrasound:

(a) Detect AV malformation
(b) Detect emboli
(c) Detect vasospasm
(d) Detect brain blood vessels stenosis

Explanation:

TRANSCRANIAL DOPPLER (TCD) ULTRASOUND

- **Low-frequency 2-MHz transducer** is used to evaluate **blood flow within** the **intracranial carotid** and **vertebrobasilar system** and the **circle of Willis**.
- **Acoustic windows**
  - Acoustic windows are naturally occurring areas of cerebral bone thin enough to allow transmission of ultrasound waves.
  - There are three commonly used acoustic windows:
    - Transtemporal
    - Transorbital
    - Transforaminal.

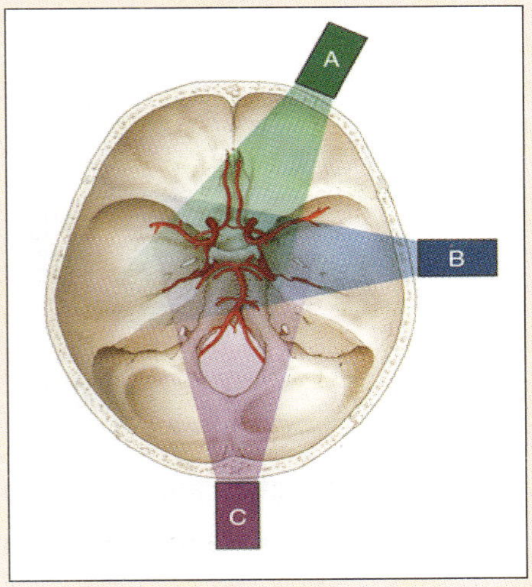

- **TCD applications** include:
  - Evaluation of intracranial stenosis and collateral circulation.
  - Detection and follow-up of vasoconstriction from subarachnoid hemorrhage.
  - Determination of brain death.
  - Evaluation of patients with sickle cell disease; and
  - Identification of arteriovenous malformation.

- TCD is **most reliable** in diagnosing stenoses of the middle cerebral artery (MCA), with sensitivities as high as 91%.
- TCD is **less reliable** for detecting stenoses of the intracranial vertebrobasilar system, anterior and posterior cerebral arteries and terminal ICA.
- Advantages of TCD ultrasound also include its availability to monitor patients in the operating room or angiographic suite for potential cerebrovascular complications.
- TCD is also capable of detecting **intraoperative microembolization**.

Ans: (d) Detect brain blood vessels stenosis

Ref: *Textbook Diagnostic Ultrasound by Rumack, 2nd Volume, 4th edition*

7. Wavelength of X-rays?

(a) 1 to 10 nm
(b) 0.1 to 10 nm
(c) 0.01 to 10 nm
(d) 0.001 to 10 nm

Explanation:

- **X-rays** are a form of **radiation** or **electromagnetic wave.**
- X-rays lie above **ultraviolet radiation**, **visible light** and **radio waves** in the spectrum, and **below cosmic radiation.**

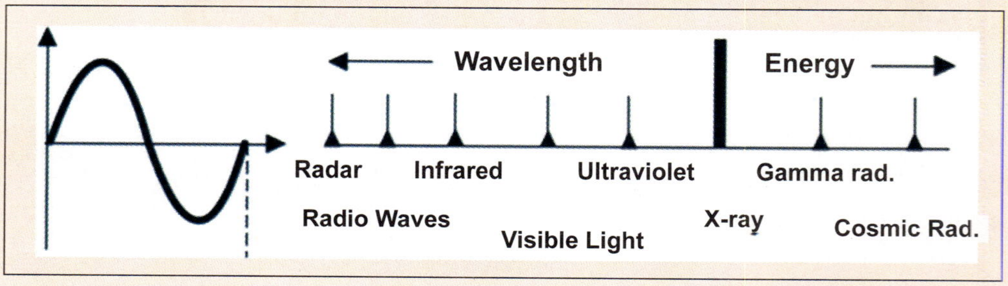

- They are a form of **high energy radiation**, with a **high frequency*** and **short wavelength***.
- When the electrons impact the target the anode X-rays are produced in two main ways:
  - Bremsstrahlung and
  - Characteristic radiation.

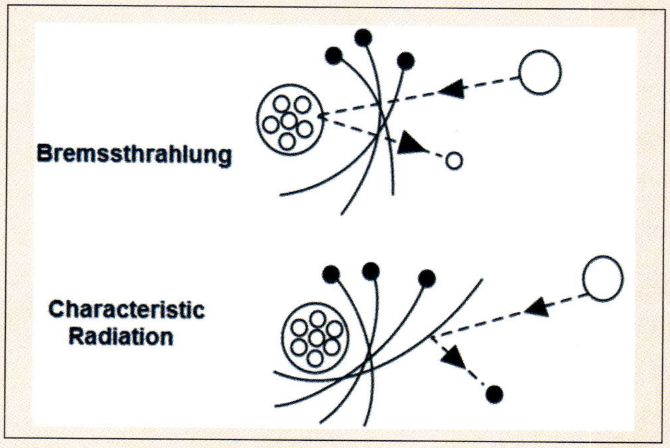

Characteristics and Properties of X-rays:

- X-rays are **electrically neutral**.

- X-rays travel in **straight lines** at the **speed of light**.
- X-rays produce biological and chemical effects.
- X-rays span a section of the electromagnetic spectrum and possess not only one frequency, but several X-rays are not visible.
- X-rays produce images on photographic film and fluorescence on certain types of crystals.
- X-rays produce secondary radiation and scattered radiation.
- Wavelength of X-rays **– 0.01 to 10 nanometers.**

Ans: (c) 0.01 to 10 nm

Ref: *Textbook Technical Fundamentals of Radiology and CT by Guillermo Avendaño*

8. Image of Chest PA Radiograph of a 30-year-old male patient. What is the most probable diagnosis?

(a) Thymoma

(b) Prevertebral abscess

(c) Lymphoma

(d) Aortic aneurysm

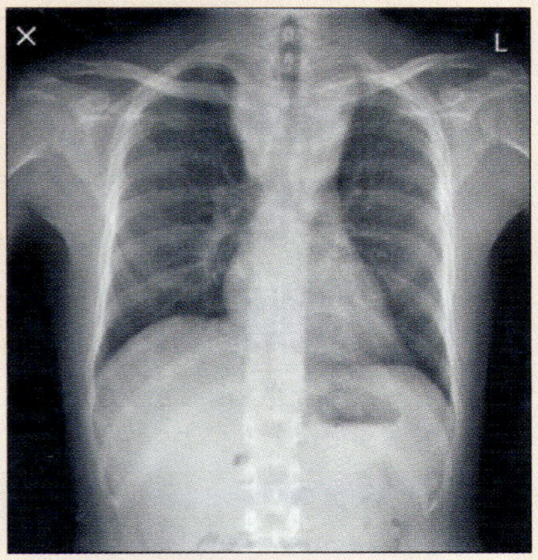

Explanation:

- The common causes of an anterosuperior mediastinal mass:
  - **Thymus**
  - **Thyroid**
  - **Thoracic aorta**
  - **Lymphoma**
  - **Teratoma**
  - **Germ cell tumours**
- On plain radiographs, **anterior mediastinal lymph node enlargement** may result in a unilateral or bilateral mediastinal abnormality.
- **Enlargement of paratracheal** or **aortopulmonary window** nodes often results in a unilateral or asymmetrical abnormality.
- Because multiple lymph nodes are involved, mediastinal masses often appear elongated or lobulated in contour. Roughly spherical masses also can be seen.
- Poor definition of the mass can indicate invasion or extension into adjacent lung.

HODGKIN'S DISEASE

- Peak incidence in the 3rd and 8th decades
- Characterized by **Reed-Sternberg** cells
- **Nodular sclerosis** cell type accounts for 50%-80% of adult cases
- Staged using **Ann Arbor system**
- **Thoracic involvement** in **85%** of cases at diagnosis
- **Lymph node involvement** in nearly all with **thoracic** involvement
- **Superior mediastinal node** enlargement in **98%**
- **Calcification of lymph nodes** common after treatment

Lung Disease

- 10% have lung involvement at diagnosis
- Nearly always associated with enlarged nodes
- Direct infiltration, lung nodules, or consolidation
- Pleural effusion in 15%, usually due to lymphatic obstruction

Ans: (c) Lymphoma

Ref: *Webb et al. Thoracic Imaging: Pulmonary and Cardiovascular Radiology, 1st edition*

9. All are USG findings in Acute Appendicitis except:

(a) Diameter greater than 6 mm (b) Non-Compressible

(c) Gut signature (d) Appendicolith

Explanation:

- **Gut signature** can be seen in both **normal and inflamed appendix**.
- The normal appendix is **compressible**, with a wall thickness of **3 mm** or less.
- The diameter of the appendix, above which acute appendicitis is highly likely, have been set at either **6 mm or 7 mm.**
- Sonographic visualization of an appendix with an **appendicolith**, regardless of **appendiceal diameter**, should also be regarded as a **positive test.**

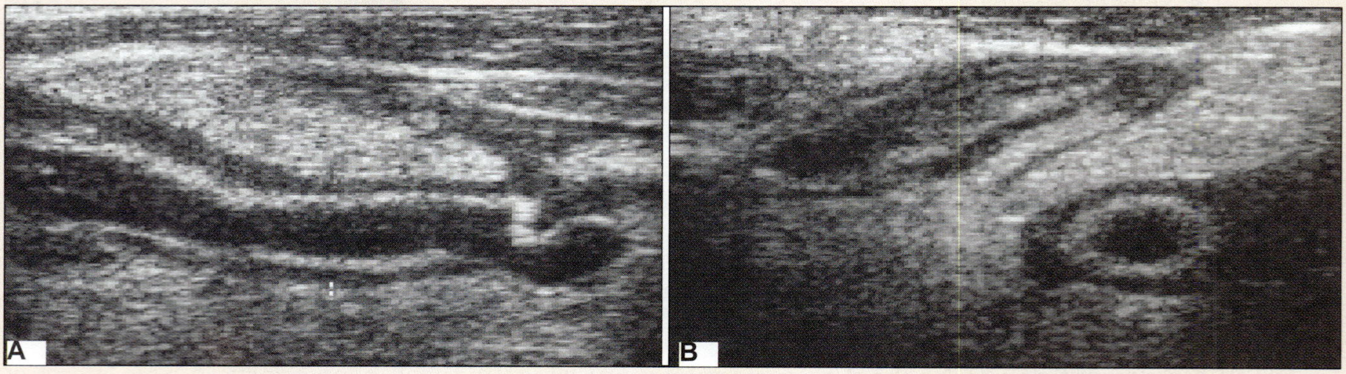

Acute appendicitis: The appendix looks **round in short axis** measures **more than 6 mm** and the **lumen is distended** with fluid. The appendix is surrounded with **inflamed fat.**

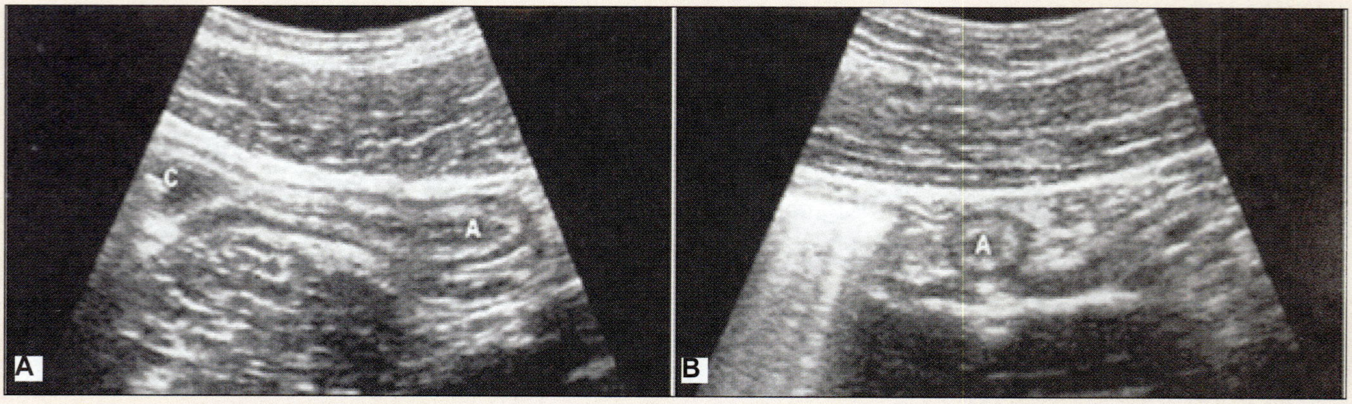

ACUTE APPENDICITIS: SONOGRAPHIC DIAGNOSIS
Patient with right lower quadrant (RLQ) pain and elevated white blood cell (WBC) count.
IDENTIFY APPENDIX
• Blind ended
• Noncompressible
• Aperistaltic tube
• Gut signature
• Arising from base of cecum
• Diameter greater than 6 mm
SUPPORTIVE FEATURES
• Inflamed perienteric fat
• Pericecal collections
• Appendicolith

SONOGRAPHY OF APPENDICEAL PERFORATION
• Loculated pericecal fluid
• Phlegmon
• Abscess
• Prominent pericecal fat
• Circumferential loss of submucosal layer of the appendix

Ans: (c) Gut signature

Ref: *Textbook Diagnostic Ultrasound by Rumack, 2nd Volume, 4th edition*

PSYCHIATRY

1. A child with obsessive compulsive disorder (OCD) undergoes imaging of brain. It is most likely to show atrophy in:

(a) Putamen (b) Cerebellum

(c) Caudate nucleus (d) Globus pallidus

Explanation:

- Structural and functional abnormalities of brain are seen in many psychiatric conditions.
- Following is the list of abnormalities found by most studies.

Condition	Structural abnormalities	Functional abnormalities
Wernicke encephalopathy	Atrophy of **mammillary bodies**	–
Marchiafava-Bignami disease	Atrophy of **corpus callosum**	–
Stimulants [Amphetamine, Cocaine]	–	Increased blood flow and activation of mesolimbic dopamine system [PET]
Inhalants	–	Increased blood flow and activation of temporal lobes [SPECT]
Schizophrenia	Enlarged **ventricles**	**Hypofrontality** {f-MRI}
Bipolar disorder	Decreased **prefrontal cortex** and cerebellar vermis Enlarged **putamen and amygdala**	–
Depression	Atrophy of **hippocampus**, **prefrontal cortex (PFC) and medial temporal lobe**	Decreased blood flow to these regions
Anxiety/Panic disorder	–	Reduction of cerebral blood flow [especially with panicogens]
PTSD	–	Hyper reactive **amygdala**
OCD	Atrophy of **caudate**	Hyperfunctioning of **insular-striatal** regions
ADHD	Smaller prefrontal cortex (PFC)	–

Ans: (c) Caudate nucleus

Ref: *Synopsis of Psychiatry, Kaplan and Saddok, 10th edition*

2. All are true regarding anorexia nervosa except:

(a) Anorexia has highest morbidity among all mental disorders

(b) Personal and social issues like pretend to people like eating

(c) BMI less than 17.5 according to DSM-5

(d) Patient won't care about weight gain

Explanation:

ANOREXIA NERVOSA

- Characterized by **intense fear of weight gain**, in spite of being low weight.
- This fear is probably due to the disturbance in the way one's body shape or weight perceived.
- This results in **restriction of food intake** especially calorie rich foods or **high carbohydrate/fatty foods**.
- **Clinical characteristics**
  - **Low weight** [BMI < 17.5]
  - **Amenorrhea***
  - **Hypoglycemia**
  - **Hypercholesterolemia***
  - **Hypo/poikilothermia***
  - **Prerenal Azotemia**
  - **Cardiac failure***
- **Biopsychosocial theories:**
  - ***Biological:*** Enlarged sulci and ventricles, blunting of diurnal Cortisol difference, lowered level of LH, FSH are noted
  - ***Psychological:*** Rejecting the greedy oral phase
  - ***Social:*** Emphasis on thinness and zero shape
- Substance use disorders, stress related disorders, mood and psychotic disorders have higher morbidity overall, not anorexia nervosa.

Ans: (a) Anorexia has highest morbidity among all mental disorders

Ref: *Synopsis of Psychiatry and Murthy RS National Mental Health Survey of India 2015-2016; Indian J Psychiatry 2017;59(1):21–26*

3. Which gene mutation is not commonly associated with Familial Alzheimer disease?

(a) Presenilin 1
(b) Presenilin 2
(c) Clusterin
(d) Amyloid precursor protein

Explanation:

- Though all the genes mentioned implicated in Alzheimer's disease, **Presenilin 1 and 2, APP** are highly correlated with familial Alzheimer's disease.
- **Clusterin** is mostly associated with **Huntington's disease***.

Alzheimer's Disease

- **Alzheimer's disease/dementia** is the most common type of dementia across the globe (In India, **Vascular dementia is most common**).
- Dementia is a chronic, progressive condition characterized by:
  - Decline in memory (Short term).
  - Executive dysfunction (Agnosia, Aphasia and Apraxia).
- While many are irreversible, some have reversible causes–alcohol, head injury, deficiency states, metabolic and endocrinopathies.

- Alzheimer's dementia is due to progressive loss of neurons starting from basal nucleus (of Meynert) which in turn due to accumulation of neurofibrillary tangles (intracellular tau proteins) and amyloid plaques (**extracellular β amyloid**) deposition.
- Since basal nucleus is the main place in brain where acetylcholine is synthesized (Ach is responsible for transferring immediate memory into short term memory), decline of memory is seen.
- *Recently, **aluminum** has been implicated for **Alzheimer's disease**.*

Cortical dementia	Sub-cortical dementia
• Memory loss is early • Aphasia is pronounced, e.g., Alzheimer's dementia	• Mood and motor symptoms first • Memory disturbance is late, e.g., Parkinson, Lewy body disease

The aim of treatment of Alzheimer's disease is preservation of existing cholinergic neurons (or at least Ach by preventing its degradation – which in turn done by inhibition of Ach-estrase).

The drugs used:

- **Ach precursors**–Choline, Lecithine.
- **AchE inhibitors**–Donapezil, Rivastigmine, Galantamine (DRG).
- **Antiglutamates**–Memantine.
- **New drugs**–Selegeline (MAOI-B type), Ondensetron, Estrogen, NSAIDs.

Also Note:

- **Clonidine** is a **central sympatholytic (α)**, used to treat **essential hypertension**, **diabetic neuropathy**, **Opioid withdrawal**, **menopausal symptoms** (**hot flushes**).

Ans: (c) Clusterin

Ref: *Harrison Textbook of Medicine*

4. Which of the following features seen in a 12-year-old child suffering from depression is not suggestive of development of bipolar disorder later?

(a) Rapid onset of depression
(b) Psychotic symptoms
(c) Mood lability
(d) Psychomotor agitation

Explanation:

- First episode of **depression** may be **unipolar or bipolar**.
- Following points will help to identify **bipolar depression** in those people without past history of **mania/hypomania:**
  - **Family history** of bipolar disorder
  - **Early onset** of depression (age)
  - **Acute onset** of depression (with or without stress)
  - **Severe** depression with **psychotic** symptoms
  - **Labile mood** (mood changes abruptly without appropriate external stimuli)
  - Psychomotor **retardation** (**Sea saw** phenomenon*).

Ans: (d) Psychomotor agitation

Ref: *Comprehensive Textbook of Psychiatry, Kaplan and Saddok*

5. Lobe atrophied in chronic schizophrenia:

(a) Frontal lobe (b) Occipital lobe
(c) Parietal lobe (d) Temporal lobe

Explanation:

- Schizophrenia is characterized by **positive and negative** symptoms.
- Several abnormalities in brain from molecular to macroscopic level have been demonstrated in these patients.
- **Hypofrontality,** i.e., **atrophy** of **frontal lobe** especially **prefrontal cortex (PFC)** is a well observed entity.
- Clinically speaking, these patients perform poorly at **frontal lobe tests**, like **Go-no go test, Stroop test, Alternate sequence test etc.**
- Historical term, **dementia precox** has been proved meaningful with new tests.

Ans: (a) Frontal lobe

Ref: *Comprehensive Textbook of Psychiatry, Kaplan and Saddok*

6. A 13-year-old victim of sexual abuse is admitted for evaluation. Which of the following factors is the least to influence in, the child developing depressive disorder in future?

(a) Negative attitude towards abuse (b) Parents with history of depression
(c) Low cognitive function (d) Abuse was penetrative

Explanation:

- The question deals with **Acute stress reaction/Post traumatic stress disorder**.
- Unusual, life/self-threatening injuries can affect the mind–resulting in negative emotions and behavioral problems.
- The causes may be natural like tsunami; man made like war and road traffic accidents; or legal like rape.
- Both victim and witness can develop these disorders.
- With respect to rape, it need not to be penetrative for a victim to develop psychological trauma.
- Others are true, i.e., those with family or past history of depression; young age; poor cognitive function (immature in colloquial sense)–increase the risk of development of ATS/PTSD.

Ans: (d) Abuse was penetrative

Ref: *Ahuja Textbook of Postgraduate Psychiatry*

7. Delusion of grandiosity is seen in all except:

(a) Schizophrenia (b) Amphetamine toxicity
(c) Frontal lobe tumour (d) Compulsive neurosis

Explanation:

Delusion

- Delusion is a **false**, **unshakable belief.**
- It is a disorder of '**content of thought**'.
- It is a **psychotic symptom** (along with hallucination, gross disturbance of speech and behaviour).

- **Bizarre delusion** means **implausible ones** (e.g., aliens following me).
- **Mood congruent delusion** are seen in **mood disorders***
  - Delusion of guilt, nihilistic delusion – **Depression**.
  - Delusion of grandeur – **Mania**.
- **Mood incongruent delusions** are characteristic of **schizophrenia*.**
- Single or few related, non-bizarre delusion seen in **delusional disorder.**
  - Delusion of infidelity: **Morbid jealousy** (Chronic alcoholics).
- For all **psychiatric disorders**, **organic** and **substance abuse** should be ruled out.
- **Frontal lobe lesions** produce **mood symptoms** (pseudo mania – orbito frontal lesion; pseudo depression – lateral frontal cortex lesion).
- **Obsessive compulsive disorder (OCD)**, a neurotic disorder, is not characterized by delusions. Obsessions are ego dystonic, whereas delusions are ego syntonic. Obsessions are not ego alien like delusion of control **(somatic passivity**).
- Note occasionally **pseudo hallucinations** can occur in **OCD***.

Ans: (d) Compulsive neurosis

Ref: *Psychiatry Made Simple by Arulvarman*

8. Drug of choice for Acute severe depression with least side effects:

(a) Mao inhibitors
(b) TCA
(c) Serotonin modulators
(d) Serotonin noradrenaline reuptake inhibitor

Explanation:

- Antidepressants are chosen based on **efficacy** and **side effects profile.**
- Out of given options, **MAO inhibitors** have several, severe side effects and not used for depression commonly.
- **TCAs**, though effective, too have significant side effects like **anti cholinergic effects** (blurring of vision, dry mouth, constipation, retention of urine) **cardiac conduction defects** etc.
- **Serotonin modulators** are new group of drugs which are yet to be proved clinically about efficacy.
- **SNRIs** are **relatively safe** among options and efficacious too.
- If SSRIs were given as option, then that would be the answer.
- Note that it takes atleast two weeks for any drug to show improvement of depressive symptoms.
- If depression is severe and patient is having high suicidal risk, then **Electroconvulsive therapy (ECT)** would be the treatment of choice.

Ans: (d) SNRI

Ref: *Are SNRIs more effective than SSRIs? A Review of the Current State of the Controversy, Psychopharmacol Bull 2008;41(2):58-85*